PREVE
SENIOR HEALTH LIBRARY

Seniors
Guide to
Good
Nutrition

By the editors of

PREVENTION
Health Books ™

RODALE

The information in this book is excerpted from *Food Smart* in the *Women's Edge Health Enhancement Guide* series (Rodale Press, 1998), *Food Smart* in the *Men's Health Life Improvement Guides* series (Rodale Press, 1996), and *Your Perfect Weight* (Rodale Press, 1995).

Cover and Interior Designer: Diane Ness Shaw

"Do You Fit This M.O.?" on page 150 was reprinted with permission from the National Osteoporosis Foundation, 1150 17th Street, NW, Suite 500, Washington, DC 20036.

"How Happy Is Your Diet?" on pages 214–15 was excerpted from *The Duke University Medical Center Book of Diet and Fitness* by Michael Hamilton, M.D.; Ronette L. Kolotkin, Ph.D.; Dianne F. Cogburn, R.D.; D. T. Moore; and Kathryn Watterson. © 1990 by Engel and Engel, Inc. Reprinted with permission of Engel and Engel, Inc., and the Duke University Diet and Fitness Center, Durham, North Carolina.

ISBN 1-57954-221-2 paperback

2 4 6 8 10 9 7 5 3 1 paperback

Contents

Part 4: Home Alone with the Refrigerator

Part 5: Your Guide to Eating Out

PREVENTION's
healthy ideas™

For the best interactive guide to healthy active
living, visit our Web site at **www.healthyideas.com**

Introduction

Eating Healthy All Life Long

It has never been easier to eat healthy. It has also never been harder.

We have more choices than our grandparents ever could have imagined. Thanks to innovations in technology and transportation, fresh fruit and vegetables are available year-round. Red meat has become decidedly leaner, and it's amazing what you can do with turkey or chicken these days.

The problem is that, despite these opportunities, many of us still live—literally—off the fat of the land. We pile on the lard-laden favorites we grew up with instead of taking full advantage of all the good things around us.

Nutritional ignorance may indeed be bliss, but it also can be deadly. We now know that eating a diet high in fruits, vegetables, and carbohydrates such as pasta and rice provides protection from cancer, heart attack, and diabetes.

Living longer is one thing, but if it means a diet of perpetual blandness, you're probably not sure it's worth it.

Neither are we. But don't worry, we're not going to tell you that you need to start some stay-at-home-with-dry-toast-and-diet-bars diet. Instead, we're going to show you how to use nutritional knowledge to make choices that will enable you to eat for pure pleasure *and* good health.

We'll tell you how to dine well when you're at a party, on a plane, in your favorite restaurant, or with the kids or grandkids at the local burger barn. We'll show you dozens of foods that will tantalize your tastebuds while battling cholesterol, migraines, and energy dips. Even better, we'll show you the right way to eat by talking about what goes on in your mind. You'll learn why you're attracted to certain foods when you're feeling lonely or stressed or depressed. Armed with that knowledge, you'll be able to choose food that won't put on pounds and harm your health.

Think of this as a book of strategies—of food smarts—that can change fundamentally the way you look at what you eat, making you not only healthier but happier.

So dig in—first to our advice, then to your new way of eating. We're sure you're going to love both your new diet and the new, healthier you!

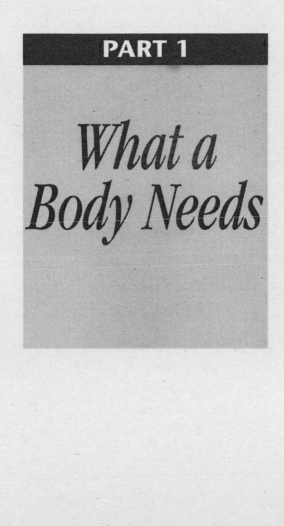

PART 1

What a Body Needs

Eat Smart for Life

Good Reasons to Make It a Habit

Whatever your age, eating right is a must for healthy living. Besides being easy, eating the right foods can do wonders for your body.

Simply by eating healthfully you can cut your risk of chronic illness—sometimes dramatically. And if you're a woman, it's doubly important to eat properly because your body undergoes extraordinary changes over the course of your lifetime. "Women menstruate, they bear children, they go through menopause," notes Joanne Curran-Celentano, R.D., Ph.D., associate professor of nutritional sciences at the University of New Hampshire in Durham. "Each one of these events puts tremendous nutritional demands on your body."

If nutrition is such a big deal, why does your doctor rarely mention it—if ever? Because for years the medical community didn't give it much value. Now research is showing the major role nutrition plays in our lives.

Those Incredible Edibles

Though scientists have barely scratched the surface in understanding the relationship between what you eat and how you feel, they've already discovered an impressive list of things that eating right can do for you. Here are some of the best.

Keep heart disease away. Heart disease ranks as the number-one cause of death in the United States. Many experts attribute this dubious distinction to a much-too-high intake of dietary fat. But they also believe that foods such as olive oil, soy, garlic, and grape juice can cut your odds of developing heart disease by nearly 25 percent.

Lower cholesterol. You probably already know that a high-fat diet can send your cholesterol level through the roof. But now there's evidence that certain foods—especially fiber-rich beans and pectin-rich fruits such as grapefruit—can help keep your cholesterol low and your arteries clear.

Reduce high blood pressure. A quartet of nutrients that you can easily get from foods—calcium, magnesium, potassium, and vitamin C—may be the nutritional tools that your body needs to help whip your blood pressure reading into shape.

Outsmart cancer. One-fourth of all breast cancers might be prevented if women cut down on dietary fat and filled up on fruits, vegetables, and whole grains.

Derail diabetes. Up to two-thirds of people with Type II (non-insulin-dependent) diabetes may very well be able to manage it simply by eating right and exercising regularly.

Beef up your bones. As many as one in two women will suffer an osteoporosis-related fracture in her lifetime. You can cut your risk in half just by making sure that you're getting enough bone-building calcium in your diet.

Eliminate weight gain. A low-fat, low-calorie eating plan that includes lots of grains and produce is your best bet for saying bye-bye to extra baggage and reducing your risk for serious health problems such as heart disease and certain types of cancer.

Turn back the clock. Many of the physical changes that occur as you get older—sagging skin, poor muscle tone, and reduced immunity—can be traced to cellular damage by renegade molecules called free radicals. Eating foods rich in antioxidants—vitamins C and E and beta-carotene—can help slow the aging process and protect against age-related disease.

Enhance immunity. Your body uses the nutrients in the food you eat to keep your immune system in good working order.

Banish fatigue. Complex carbohydrates such as whole grains, beans, and vegetables can help keep your energy level on an even keel. Just as important, they supply the nutrients your body needs most when it's tired or run-down.

Defuse stress. Many experts believe that prolonged stress depletes your internal supplies of key nutrients such as calcium and zinc. There's also preliminary evidence that vitamin C can help protect your body against the effects of stress.

Influence your emotions. Your body uses substances in food to produce neurotransmitters, brain chemicals that dramatically affect your mood. So what you eat can lift your spirits—or bring you down.

Boost your brainpower. You can turbocharge your mental alertness, concentration, and memory by munching on a little bit of low-fat protein. Protein supports the production of neurotransmitters that keep you mentally sharp.

Minimize the symptoms of menopause. Women in Japan experience fewer menopausal symp-
(continued on page 8)

Cholesterol: A Family Affair?

Since childhood, Carol Politi, an administrative associate at a Pennsylvania bank, and her identical twin sister had allergies and skin problems. During adulthood, they were plagued with respiratory problems and exhaustion. But it wasn't until a health crisis hit her 5-year-old daughter that Carol made drastic changes to her family's eating habits. The effects on her own health were positively astounding. Here's her story.

A fat-loving, cigarette-smoking couch potato—that's the type of person you probably think of as having high cholesterol. So when my lively, petite, 5-year-old was diagnosed with dangerously high cholesterol, I was understandably shocked. Even though my twin sister and I have been plagued with high cholesterol and other health problems all our lives, I never thought such a problem could hit my child—and at such a young age. My motherly instincts to do everything to protect her health were jolted into action.

The first thing I did was throw away all the junk food in our house. It was quickly followed by eggs, hamburgers, and ice cream. To get my daughter to eat right, I knew the whole family's diet had to change. I started serving lots of fish, chicken, and pasta. Vegetables and fruits, never big in our household, became the house staples. I started making my own low-fat cookies and chips so my children could still snack on something salty or sweet. Occasionally, we would allow ourselves a fast-food meal or a slice of iced cake.

Thankfully, the dietary changes had an immediate positive effect on Christina's cholesterol. But after 3 months, I also discovered something more: a remarkable change in my own health. After lifelong bouts with upper respiratory problems from allergies, I hadn't had a sniffle. My skin, usually cracked and dry or itchy with rashes, was smooth and clear. My cholesterol dropped from 244 to 190. And, while I wasn't looking, 25 pounds just melted off me. At some point, my energy level soared. I tackled the responsibilities of my job and family with newfound stamina.

It has been 2 years since I pruned the fat from my diet, and I've never been healthier. I've missed 3 days of work over this period, a far cry from my record 25 days during one allergy season. Interestingly, I have a built-in measure of success: my identical twin sister. She continued to eat fat-laden foods during my 2-year transformation, and her allergies and skin problems persisted. Fortunately, she's found inspiration in my story, and she's beginning to make healthy lifestyle changes. I'll be there every step of the way to help. They say that there are two sides to every story. I'm counting on these two stories to come out the same.

toms and side effects than women in the United States. Researchers think that they know why: Japanese cuisine relies heavily on soy foods, which contain phytoestrogens, plant compounds that act much like estrogen in the body.

Protect your skin. Eating healthfully can help prevent acne, canker sores, hives, and other minor skin eruptions. There's evidence, too, that munching lots of fruits and vegetables can make you less likely to develop skin cancer.

Prevent anemia. Anemia, a condition usually characterized by extreme fatigue, results from a shortage of iron in the blood. You can replenish your iron stores by eating foods such as lean meats and kidney beans.

Vanquish varicose veins. A high-fiber diet, combined with regular exercise, can prevent constipation and weight gain, both of which can lead to varicose veins.

Protect your teeth. Calcium, your body's main bone-builder, keeps teeth healthy and strong. Vitamin C and folate also chip in, feeding the gums and helping to ward off infection.

Good Health by the Plateful

You'll reap all these benefits—and more—when you eat smart. In the pages that follow, we lay out for you a comprehensive nutrition strategy that you can customize to fit your needs and lifestyle. You'll get expert advice on virtually every aspect of shaping and maintaining a healthy diet—from navigating a salad bar to cooking with herbs and spices; from ordering Chinese takeout to curing a craving for chocolate.

Yes, you'll have to make some adjustments in

Why Not Just a Multivitamin?

While taking a multivitamin is good nutritional insurance, it won't provide all the nutrients you need. A perfect example is calcium. While it is often added to multivitamins, the amount is usually only a fraction of the Daily Value because calcium isn't easily compacted like some vitamins or minerals. You would have to take a pill about three times larger than an average multivitamin to get all that you need, according to Abby Bloch, R.D., Ph.D., coordinator of clinical nutrition research at Memorial Sloan-Kettering Hospital in New York City.

Also, your body needs things that a pill can't deliver, such as complex carbohydrates, protein, and fiber.

Multivitamins can't provide more than a few phytonutrients—those naturally occurring chemical compounds that we can get from fruits and vegetables. A well-known example of phytonutrients is the carotenoids. There are about 600 different carotenoids, many of which protect against disease, particularly cancer and heart disease. But only one, beta-carotene, is commonly found in supplements.

Another concern with relying solely on a multivitamin is your body's ability to absorb and use nutrients. Vitamins and minerals in supplements need to be extracted from foods or made synthetically, and this can make them harder for your body to absorb. (Iron, which is especially important as we age, is a good example of this.)

your current eating habits. But we promise that they're painless. In fact, as you switch to our healthy way of eating, you may find that you can eat more than ever and still be fit and healthy!

So get set to dig in. You're going to love what good nutrition can do for you.

Low-Fat Is First

Get Your Nutrients in the Right Ratios

When you get right down to it, food is energy, pure and simple. It fuels your body by supplying it with calories to burn. You can consume and burn those calories in one of three forms: carbohydrates, protein, or fat.

Ideally, we should get about 60 to 65 percent of our calories from carbohydrates, about 10 percent from protein, and the remaining 25 to 30 percent from fat. This is close to the nutritional profile that studies around the world have linked to lower rates of heart disease and cancer. In reality, most Americans are falling quite short of this mark.

By one estimate, the typical person consumes just 20 to 25 percent of calories from carbohydrates—less than half the recommended amount. That means, of course, that we're making up the difference by over-doing it on protein and fat. And how! Statistics suggest that we're eating roughly twice as much protein as we should, with fat tipping the scales at 34 percent of calories.

Certainly, these days we're much more fat-conscious than we used to be, and that's good. Eating low-fat is important. "But we have to remember that diets are about more than just fat," says Doris Derelian, R.D., Ph.D., former president of the American Dietetic Association. They're about balance—getting healthful amounts of not only fat but carbohydrates and protein, too.

Carbs: The Tiger in Your Tank

Of all three nutrients, carbohydrates are your body's fuel of choice. They easily break down into a form that your body uses to keep its systems running smoothly and efficiently. They also team up with protein, forming compounds that are essential for combating infections, lubricating joints, and maintaining healthy skin, bones, and nails.

Actually, there are two kinds of carbohydrates, and your body utilizes them in slightly different ways. Simple carbohydrates consist of tiny, single or double molecules of sugar. They have familiar names, like glucose, fructose, and lactose. These carbs are already in their most basic form, which means that they are absorbed into the bloodstream quite quickly. There they circulate as glucose, or blood sugar, until getting snapped up by cells and converted into energy.

Simple carbohydrates also join together to form complex carbohydrates. Complex carbs are found almost exclusively in plant foods such as grains, beans, fruits, and vegetables. When you eat complex carbohydrates, your digestive system has to break them down into their simple form before they can be absorbed into your bloodstream and used as fuel. This "production time" makes for a steadier, longer-lasting energy source than simple carbs provide.

In fact, there's evidence to suggest that your body burns more calories digesting complex carbohydrates than digesting protein or fat. Research has shown that vegetarians have higher metabolic rates than meat eaters, and scientists attribute the difference to the vegetarians' high-carbohydrate diets.

If you're following a 2,000-calorie-a-day eating plan, you should get about 1,200 of those calories as carbs. That translates to about 300 grams of carbohydrate per day.

We consume far fewer complex carbohydrates than we should—and far fewer than we used to. At the beginning of the twentieth century, carbohydrate consumption in the United States hovered around a much healthier 70 percent of calories. Ironically, as we got wealthier, our eating habits got worse, as meats and sweets, which were symbols of affluence, became more affordable, says Maria Linder, Ph.D., professor of biochemistry at California State University, Fullerton.

So what can you do to get your carbohydrate intake on track? Give these tips a try.

Stay whole. Whole-grain foods such as brown rice, whole-wheat bread, and oatmeal are better carbohydrate choices than refined foods, says Nan Kathryn Fuchs, Ph.D., a nutritionist in Sebastopol, California, and nutrition editor of *Women's Health Letter*. Refined grains such as enriched white flour and white rice are missing some B-complex vitamins, which are essential to carbohydrate metabolism. They also don't have fiber to ensure that your body absorbs carbohydrates at a slow, steady pace.

Read the fine print. Check the label on whole-wheat bread to make sure that whole-wheat flour, not just wheat flour, tops the ingredients list, Dr. Fuchs advises. You can't go by the color of the bread—some manufacturers add coloring to their breads and other baked goods to make them look browner and more wholesome.

Pair off pasta. Spaghetti, macaroni, noodles, and other types of pasta are usually made from white flour, so they're not as good a carbohydrate source as whole grains. Improve their nutritional profile by topping them with carb-rich veggies, Dr. Fuchs suggests. For example, add lightly steamed broccoli or escarole, red and green peppers, onions, garlic, mushrooms, zucchini, or any vegetable you like to traditional red sauce.

Foil the fat. Croissants, biscuits, many crackers, potato and corn chips, French fries, and processed macaroni and cheese contain more calories from fat than from carbohydrates. The same goes for packaged rice pilaf dishes, potatoes au gratin, and some breakfast cereals—especially granola. If you must eat these foods, reserve them for an occasional treat, Dr. Fuchs recommends.

Protein: Too Much of a Good Thing?

You might think of protein as the Swiss Army knife of nutrients. Your body uses it to carry out an astounding array of tasks. Indeed, every single cell in your body contains protein. It plays an indispensable role in building and repairing body tissues, digesting food, and fighting infections. It supports the manufacture of chemical messengers in your brain and makes you more mentally alert. In a pinch, it can be converted to fuel.

Chemically, proteins consist of varying combinations of about 20 amino acids. Your body can produce most of these amino acids, but there are nine essential ones that it can get only from the foods you eat. Lysine falls into this category. Your body needs it in order to absorb calcium, the mineral that keeps your bones strong.

Red meats and dairy products were once considered superior protein sources because most contain all of the essential amino acids—in other words, they're complete proteins. Their down side, of course, is that they also contain large amounts of heart-unhealthy saturated fat.

Plant foods such as grains, beans, fruits, and vegetables are incomplete proteins, meaning that individually, they don't supply all of the essential amino acids. But you can make them complete by combining them.

Even better, it's not necessary to eat these complementary foods at the same time to reap the benefits of a complete protein. Thanks to the rather leisurely pace of the digestive process, the oatmeal you eat for breakfast combines with the baked beans you eat for lunch, the sunflower seeds you have for a snack, and the rice you eat for dinner to create a high-quality protein that has all of the essential amino acids.

The Daily Value for protein is 50 grams. But you shouldn't worry too much about not getting enough protein. Studies indicate that most people get more than enough. When you eat more protein than your body can use, the excess is stored as body fat. It can also interfere with the absorption of some minerals, such as calcium.

You can get all the protein you need without fear of overdoing it. Just heed this advice from the experts.

Minimize meat. Change the way you look at your dinner plate. Relegate meat to a bit part and let grains, beans, fruits, and vegetables take over the starring role. This dietary recasting supplies a sufficient amount of protein, while sparing you unwanted saturated fat and cholesterol. "If we planned our meals around plant foods instead of meat, we'd be much better off," says Elizabeth Somer, R.D., author of *Nutrition for Women* and *Food and Mood*.

Visit your local fishmonger. Broiled, baked, or poached, fish is a standout source of protein that is also low in saturated fat. As a bonus, fish such as salmon, mackerel, and tuna contain omega-3 fatty acids, which may help protect against heart disease.

Love those legumes. Nutrition-wise, dried beans and peas in all their different colors and shapes have plenty going for them. Of course, they contain generous amounts of protein: One-half cup of kidney beans, for example, has more protein than either a whole egg or 2 tablespoons of chunky peanut butter.

Celebrate soy. Tofu, tempeh, and other soy foods offer abundant supplies of plant protein. Technically, soy is a legume. But it merits special mention because it is also rich in phytoestrogens, chemical compounds that may reduce the risk of breast cancer. Soy foods are so versatile that you can use them as healthy substitutes for high-fat ingredients in everything from meat loaf to cheesecake.

Fat: Get the Facts

You probably already know all the bad stuff about fat: It clogs your arteries, sets the stage for heart disease, magnifies your risk of certain types of cancer, and ups your odds of gallstones and osteoporosis-related frac-

Don't Get Caught in the Fat Trap

You ate an entire package of your favorite fat-free fig bars in just 1 day, but you're not too worried. After all, they're fat-free.

Fat-free, yes. Calorie-free, no. While you may not have consumed a smidgen of fat, you've already downed a whopping 1,200 calories—almost an entire day's allotment spent on your fig-bar fling.

With all the emphasis on fat these days, and with so many nonfat and low-fat products available, many of us have gotten the impression that we no longer need to watch our calorie intakes. But calories do still count. And it takes just 3,500 of them to add another pound on you.

The next time you're tempted to eat the whole thing, refer to these figures for a jolt back to calorie reality.

---

tures. With a rap sheet like that, fat doesn't figure to be the kind of dietary company you'd want to keep. Yet it's absolutely essential to your good health.

"We spend a lot of time trying to get rid of the fat in our diets," says Michele Trankina, Ph.D., nutritional physiologist and professor of biological sciences at St. Mary's University in San Antonio. "In reality, our bodies need a certain percentage of the nutrient to function properly."

Fat is an internal transportation system, moving fat-soluble vitamins A, D, E, and K to their job sites within your body. It surrounds vital organs such as your heart and kidneys, protecting them from injury. It maintains body temperature, insulates nerves, and

Snack	Calories per Serving	Calories per Package
Fat-free caramel corn cakes	50	700
Fat-free chocolate cookie cakes	50	600
Fat-free fig bars	100	1,200
Low-fat tortilla chips	110	880
Pretzel chips	110	880
Reduced-fat mini cheese crackers	120	600
Reduced-fat mini chocolate chip cookies	130	910

supports the production of compounds that regulate blood pressure, blood clotting, and inflammation.

Your body also uses fat to store calories until they're needed for energy. In fact, of all three nutrients, fat is the most efficient at this task. It can hold 9 calories per gram, compared with protein and carbohydrates' four.

There are actually three types of fat found in foods. Of the trio, monounsaturated and polyunsaturated fat are considered the healthiest. Studies have shown that vegetable oils rich in monounsaturates (such as canola and olive oils) and polyunsaturates (such as corn and soybean oils) can help lower your total cholesterol count. And, as mentioned, omega-3 fatty acids, polyunsaturated fats found in some types of fish, have similar heart-healthy effects.

On the other hand, high amounts of saturated fat—the kind found in meat and dairy products—have been linked to an increased risk of heart disease and colon cancer.

So just how low should you go with your fat consumption? Many experts recommend 25 percent of calories from fat. Based on a 2,000-calorie-a-day diet, no more than 500 calories should come from fat. And since there are 9 calories in 1 gram of fat, you'd want to limit yourself to about 55 grams of fat a day.

Thankfully, managing your fat intake doesn't require perpetual number crunching. The following strategies take the hassle out of low-fat living.

Think in thirds. The American Heart Association has devised the Rule of Thirds: One-third of daily fat grams from monounsaturates, up to one-third from polyunsaturates, and no more than one-third from saturates. If you eat 2,000 calories and 55 grams of fat a day, no more than 18 grams (one-third of the grams of fat) should come from saturated fat.

Oust the obvious. Scan your diet for easy ways to trim fat. For example, you can bake, steam, broil, or microwave your foods rather than frying them, says Elaine Kvitka-Nevins, R.D., a nutrition consultant in Scottsdale, Arizona. Spread your morning toast with all-fruit preserves instead of butter. Switch from full-fat ice cream to low-fat or nonfat ice cream or frozen yogurt. "There are a million ways to cut your fat intake," she says.

Beyond Calcium and Iron

Eight Essential Vitamins and Minerals

Pick a fruit. Any fresh, ripe fruit will do—cantaloupe or cherries, papaya or peach. Now take a bite. Suddenly your mouth is awash with flavor as the juices drench every square millimeter of your tongue. Ambrosial bursts tantalize your palate as you chew. *Mmmm . . .* delicious.

Your tastebuds thank you for this gustatory indulgence. And the rest of your body seconds the motion. Of course, your tastebuds are only interested in the sensuous pleasure that eating provides. The rest of your body has much more at stake. It relies on food for vitamins and minerals, substances you need to survive and thrive.

Feed Your Body Right

Your body uses about two dozen vitamins and minerals every day just to support routine bodily functions, explains Cheryl Rock, Ph.D., professor of nutrition at the University of Michigan in Ann Arbor. Two of these nutrients—vitamin D and vitamin K—it can make itself. The rest must come from foods.

Unfortunately, many people, particularly women,

Do You Need Supplements?

Experts agree that the best way to get your vitamins and minerals is by eating right. But sometimes specific health or lifestyle issues make it difficult to get the nutrients your body requires through diet alone. In those instances, you may want to consider taking a supplement to pick up the slack.

Use the following questions as a guide to determine where you might be falling short, nutrient-wise. Before you begin a supplement program, though, it's a good idea to talk to your doctor or a qualified nutrition expert.

Do you smoke cigarettes or have you recently quit? Smoking appears to deplete vitamin C stores.

Are you at high risk for heart disease? Vitamin E may help keep your heart healthy.

Do you consume dairy products such as skim milk, low-fat or nonfat yogurt, and low-fat cheese? These are some of the best sources of bone-building calcium. If they're not on your menu, you may not be getting enough of the mineral.

Do you eat meat? If you don't eat at least three 3-ounce servings of red meat a week, you might benefit from an iron supplement.

Have you passed through menopause? Folate is important for you, too—it can reduce your risk of heart disease and cervical cancer.

aren't very good at getting their daily share of essential nutrients. The problem for women stems, in part, from low calorie intakes. The average woman eats roughly 1,800 calories a day—maybe less in the middle of a diet. By comparison, when dietitians at Utah State University in Logan tried to design a menu that supplied adequate amounts of all the vitamins and minerals that women need, they couldn't get the calorie count below 2,200.

What's more, women's bodies require more of certain nutrients than men's do. For example, both pregnancy and menopause can boost a woman's daily calcium quota by as much as 50 percent. Yet most women don't get nearly enough of the mineral to begin with.

In fact, calcium is one of eight nutrients that women need in their diets, says Margo Woods, D.Sc., who teaches nutrition at Tufts University School of Medicine in Boston. The other seven? Well, you've probably already guessed iron. Then there are the antioxidants—beta-carotene and vitamins C and E—plus folate, vitamin B_6, and zinc.

How Much Is Enough?

Take a look at the nutrition information on any packaged food, and you'll see the abbreviation DV. It stands for Daily Value, a federal government label guideline for how much of a certain nutrient you should be getting each day. There are DVs established for 25 vitamins and minerals as well as for other nutrients, including carbohydrates, protein, and fat.

What the label doesn't tell you is that the DVs do not reflect a woman's unique nutritional needs. The recommended intakes for the various vitamins and minerals are, for the most part, based on the nutrient requirements of a 15- to 18-year-old male.

Far more useful for women are the Recommended Dietary Allowances, or RDAs. (The exceptions are folate, vitamin E, and calcium, for which the DVs are considered better guidelines.) The RDAs take

Diet Soda Dive-Bombs Calcium

Elizabeth, age 43, considers herself a healthy eater. She eats a bagel with jam for breakfast, a salad or turkey sandwich for lunch, and pasta or fish—no red meat!—with plenty of vegetables for dinner. She snacks on sunflower seeds, raisins, pretzels, and fruit. Her fave is low-fat frozen yogurt. And for liquids, nothing with calories passes her lips—ever. Her drink of choice is diet cola, which she buys by the case. As she approaches menopause, she wonders, "Am I getting adequate nutrients?"

Annette Pederson, R.D., dietitian and health educator at the Diabetes Care and Education Center of Robinson Memorial Hospital in Ravenna, Ohio, says, "It sounds like she eats a well-balanced diet that includes a variety of foods." Thanks to her polite refusal of any beverages beyond water and diet soda, however, her diet is sorely lacking in calcium—a mineral crucial to a woman approaching menopause and its accompanying risk of osteoporosis.

What's more, carbonated beverages, including diet colas, contain phosphoric acid, which is bad news. Studies have found that one or two diet colas a day contain enough phosphoric acid to interfere with calcium absorption. Unless Elizabeth cuts down on colas and includes more dairy products in her diet, she could be setting herself up for osteoporosis.

into account gender, age, and whether you are pregnant or nursing. Currently, RDAs are established for 11 vitamins and 7 minerals, plus protein. And they're updated periodically, as research turns up new information about how much of a nutrient is required to correct a deficiency and how much is normally consumed by people in good health.

Still, some experts contend that even the RDAs don't make the grade as dietary standards. First, while the RDAs will pretty much guarantee that you will keep deficiency at bay, they aren't a measure of how much you need for optimum health. Second, the RDAs are set to meet the needs of *healthy* people; people trying to fight disease need more.

Take vitamin C as an example. The RDA (and the DV) for women is 60 milligrams. Yet many studies of the nutrient show that vitamin C does the most good—functioning as an antihistamine, boosting immunity, and protecting against cancer—in daily doses of at least a few hundred milligrams.

To reap all the health benefits that vitamins and minerals offer, you may have to go beyond the RDAs (while remaining within safe limits).

The Essential Eight

For many women, just meeting the minimum daily requirement is a tall order—never mind getting extra. To help make it easier, here's a rundown of the eight nutrients that you need most, along with their recommended daily intakes and best food sources. Where appropriate, we've asked several experts to recommend protective amounts that may help ward off disease.

Calcium: The Best for Your Bones
By now you probably know that calcium reigns as your body's champion bone-builder. The mineral joins forces with phosphorus to form hard, crystal-like substances that provide the framework for a strong skeleton.

Around age 40, you begin to lose calcium from your bones faster than it can be replaced. This process speeds up at menopause as production of estrogen—which helps your bones absorb calcium—shifts into low gear.

In the Netherlands, a team of scientists evaluating 33 studies of a total of 4,000 18- to 50-year-old women concluded that those who consume 1,000 milligrams of calcium a day retain 1 percent more bone in their hips and backs every year than those who don't get that much. So a 40-year-old woman who starts defending her current calcium stores may have preserved 20 percent more of her bone density by the time she reaches age 60. This could make the difference between a sturdy skeleton and a brittle one.

Calcium can do more for you than keep your bones strong. One study of almost 35,000 women concluded that those with the highest calcium intakes have half the risk of heart disease–related death of those with the lowest calcium intakes. There's also evidence that the mineral can minimize premenstrual and menstrual symptoms such as breast tenderness, cramps, and backaches, and can cut your chances of developing kidney stones.

Calcium is at its best only when it's working with vitamin D. Without D to guide it, calcium can't break through the intestinal wall to get where it wants to go. Fortunately, your body makes plenty of D on its own—with a little help from Old Sol. Sunlight is a natural source of D. Because vitamin D is toxic in large amounts, it should never be taken in supplemental form.

How much you need: The National Institutes of Health recommend that women between the ages of 25 and 50 get 1,000 milligrams of calcium a day. Experts say you may need as much as 1,200 to 1,500 milligrams a day for maximum health benefits. As for vitamin D, you should aim for the RDA for women of 5 micrograms, or 200 international units (IU).

Where to get it: Fortified skim milk can supply healthy doses of both calcium and vitamin D. An 8-ounce glass contains 302 milligrams of calcium. (You'll need to check the label for the vitamin D content. Milk is often fortified with 100 IU per cup.) Other good food sources of calcium include nonfat yogurt, nonfat or low-fat cheese, canned salmon with bones, calcium-fortified orange juice, and collard greens.

Iron: The Mineral for Mettle

True or false: Women must take supplements of iron to make up for what's lost during menstruation.

True . . . and false.

Yes, you lose iron every month via your period. But many experts agree that few women need supplements to replenish what's lost. In general, we get plenty of iron in our diets. Those who stand the greatest chance of running low are women who have heavy periods and female athletes who train vigorously.

Still, roughly 20 percent of all women don't get as much iron as they should. "I would say that women need to be a little more thoughtful than men about iron, in the same way that women should be a little more cautious about their calcium intakes because of osteoporosis," says Adria Sherman, Ph.D., professor and chair of the department of nutritional sciences at Rutgers University in New Brunswick, New Jersey.

Iron's primary responsibility in your body is the formation of hemoglobin, the substance that helps your red blood cells transport oxygen from your lungs to the rest of your body. It also helps prepare your immune system's infection-fighters for battle and supports the production of collagen to build your body's tissues.

When you don't get enough iron or your body's stores run low, the red blood cells can't move oxygen as they should. This can lead to fatigue, pallor, and listlessness, which are all hallmarks of iron-deficiency anemia, Dr. Sherman says.

How much you need: The RDA of iron for premenopausal women is 15 milligrams a day. That's roughly one-third more than you'll need at menopause. (The DV is 18 milligrams.)

Where to get it: Foods supply two kinds of iron. Heme iron, found primarily in meats, is better absorbed than nonheme iron, found primarily in plant foods such as potatoes and kale. But you can improve the absorption rate by pairing off a nonheme iron source with a vitamin C source. For example, if you're having a bowl of Cream of Wheat for breakfast, add a glass of vitamin C–rich orange juice to your meal.

If you prefer meat as your iron source, choose a lean cut such as bottom or top round. Even chicken or turkey breast can boost iron. Or add a little ham to baked beans to enhance the absorption of iron from the beans.

Beta-Carotene: Color Yourself Healthy

Technically, beta-carotene is not a vitamin. It is a member of the carotenoid family, a group of compounds that give red, orange, and yellow fruits and vegetables their hues. So why mention it here? Because your body converts beta-carotene into vitamin A on an as-needed basis.

Vitamin A plays a major role in the development and maintenance of your immune system. Without it, you'd become more vulnerable to a host of infectious diseases, from measles to AIDS. Vitamin A also protects your vision and supports bodily processes such as growth and cell differentiation.

But too much vitamin A is not a good thing. In large amounts, it can poison your system and produce severe symptoms, including anemia and an enlarged liver and spleen. These problems are more likely to be caused by supplements than by foods. Most experts recommend that you get your vitamin A from beta-carotene, since you essentially can't overdose on the nutrient. And preliminary studies have shown that eating lots of beta-carotene-rich fruits and vegetables can greatly reduce your risk of heart disease, cancer, and stroke.

For example, among 87,000 participants in the Harvard University Nurses' Health Study—considered a landmark study in the women's health field—women who ate 15 to 21 milligrams of beta-carotene a day were 22 percent less likely to have heart attacks than women who ate less than 6 milligrams a day. Those with high beta-carotene intakes also had a 40 percent lower risk of stroke.

Another study showed that eating foods rich in beta-carotene cut women's odds of developing breast cancer after menopause by more than half. The women's risk dropped off sharply with a daily beta-carotene intake of about 4 milligrams—the amount in a little less than one-third of a carrot.

Beta-carotene also plays a role in protecting against cervical dysplasia, a condition involving the development of abnormal cells in the cervix that can progress to cancer. There's evidence that women who don't get enough beta-carotene in their diets are more likely to have cervical dysplasia.

(continued on page 30)

27

Put a Little Meat on Your Bones

Fifty years ago, few of us would have served a meal without a slab of sirloin or a hunk of ham. But these days, it seems we're going meatless—or almost meatless—in droves, believing a vegetarian or semivegetarian lifestyle is key to good health.

Indeed, an array of studies have linked vegetarianism to a reduced risk of atherosclerosis (clogging of the arteries) and high blood pressure, both major contributors to heart disease. Other preliminary research suggests that a meatless diet may protect against cancer, prevent osteoporosis, and minimize menopausal symptoms such as hot flashes, insomnia, and weight gain.

The downside is, cutting down on meat cuts back on a top-notch source of certain essential nutrients. Take iron, a mineral that 40 percent of women chronically run low on. You won't find a better food source of it than red meat, says Elizabeth Somer, R.D., author of *Nutrition for Women* and *Food and Mood*. She points out that your body can absorb up to three times as much iron from meat as from plant foods such as vegetables, fruits, legumes, and grains.

Some experts like Somer recommend that people eat some meat every day—maybe a couple of ounces mixed into chili or a stir-fry. But if you'd really rather go without, experts say you should pay particular attention to your intakes of the following nutrients.

28

Iron. Many plant foods have an abundance of iron, but it's nonheme iron, the kind that isn't absorbed into your bloodstream all that easily. To make up for that, consume whole grains, beans, and leafy green vegetables. If you think you're running low, eat iron-rich foods with vitamin C–rich foods. Vitamin C can help your body hang on to more iron.

Vitamin B_{12}. Vegetarians who eschew not only meat, fish, and poultry but also eggs and dairy products are at considerable risk for running low on vitamin B_{12}, since it's almost exclusively available in foods from animal sources. An ongoing shortage of the nutrient can lead to pernicious anemia, which is sometimes fatal. Get this B vitamin by consuming lots of B_{12}-fortified foods such as breakfast cereals and B_{12}-fortified soy milk, or by taking a B_{12} supplement.

Calcium. Vegetarians who don't consume dairy products need to keep an eye on their calcium intakes. Connie Weaver, Ph.D., professor of foods and nutrition at Purdue University in West Lafayette, Indiana, recommends getting as much calcium as you can from foods—particularly dark, leafy greens and nuts—and making up the difference with a supplement. Or try a calcium-fortified beverage such as soy milk or orange juice.

Scientists attribute beta-carotene's preventive powers to the fact that it's an antioxidant, which means it works primarily by neutralizing free radicals, harmful molecules that damage healthy molecules by robbing them of electrons (a process known as oxidation). Free radicals occur naturally in your body as by-products of day-to-day functions. But their numbers grow dramatically in the presence of external factors such as air pollution, cigarette smoke, and excessive sun exposure.

You have good reason to choose beta-carotene-rich foods over supplements. These foods contain other members of the carotenoid clan, including alpha-carotene, lycopene, zeaxanthin, and lutein. Preliminary research suggests that these compounds have disease-fighting potential as well. In fact, they may turn out to be even more potent than beta-carotene itself.

How much you need: No RDA or DV has been established for beta-carotene. But to meet the RDA of vitamin A for women, which is 800 micrograms retinol equivalents (the DV is 5,000 IU), you'd have to take in about 5 milligrams of beta-carotene a day. Some experts recommend a much higher dosage—15 to 20 milligrams (25,000 to 33,000 IU)—to obtain beta-carotene's disease-fighting effects.

Where to get it: The best sources of beta-carotene have deep, rich colors. Check out red, orange, and yellow produce such as carrots, cantaloupe, and sweet potatoes, and dark green, leafy vegetables such as turnip greens, beet greens, spinach, and parsley.

Folate: Not Just Baby Food

When you look in the mirror, you can thank folate for what you see. This B vitamin helps to make you . . .

you. It works with about 20 different enzymes to construct DNA, the material that contains your very own genetic code.

Scientists say that folate plays a significant role in the health of developing babies. Study after study has shown that the vitamin can protect against life-threatening defects of the brain and spine, such as spina bifida. These problems, known as neural tube defects, occur during the first 2 weeks of pregnancy—long before most women realize that they've conceived. That's why it's so important for all women of childbearing age to make sure that they're getting enough of the nutrient in their diets.

"Fifty to 70 percent (of neural tube defects) could be prevented if women got enough folate," says Joanne Curran-Celentano, R.D., Ph.D., associate professor of nutritional sciences at the University of New Hampshire in Durham.

But according to one survey, a startling 90 percent of women of reproductive age don't know that folate can protect the health of unborn babies. And 85 percent are unaware of the U.S. Public Health Service recommendation that all women capable of bearing children get 400 micrograms of folate every day. Most of us get only half of that amount.

Even if pregnancy isn't in the picture, don't shirk folate—it's essential to your good health, too. For starters, it helps to keep your cardiovascular system in tip-top shape by clearing it of homocysteine, a bad-guy amino acid that research has linked to heart disease and stroke. Apparently, folate speeds the metabolism of homocysteine into a less harmful substance, so it can't do your arteries any harm.

One review of all the published studies on the

subject concluded that increasing folate intake to 400 micrograms a day could prevent as many as 50,000 heart disease–related deaths every year. This means the average woman's heart disease risk could drop by more than 6 percent.

Folate may also help protect against cervical cancer. In a study at the University of Alabama in Birmingham, researchers found that women with high folate levels in their cervical cells were two to five times less likely than women with low folate levels to develop dysplasia when exposed to risk factors such as cigarette smoke, human papillomavirus, and contraceptives.

If you take oral contraceptives, be aware that they can deplete your body's stores of folate and the other B vitamins, according to Chris Rosenbloom, R.D., Ph.D., associate professor in the department of nutrition and dietetics at Georgia State University in Atlanta and a spokesperson for the American Dietetic Association.

How much you need: The U.S. Public Health Service advises—and many experts agree—that you should try for at least 400 micrograms a day. (The DV is 0.4 milligram, or 400 micrograms; the RDA for women is 180 micrograms.) "But your body can use only about 50 percent of the folate that you consume," says Shirley A. A. Beresford, Ph.D., an epidemiologist at the University of Washington in Seattle. "So to get 400 micrograms of folate a day, you'd have to take in roughly 800 micrograms." A multivitamin can help you hit the mark.

Where to get it: Recognizing the importance of folate in the diet, the Food and Drug Administration requires that certain grain-based foods manufactured in the United States—including pastas, cereals, and breads—be fortified with folate. Read the labels of the products you choose to find out their folate contents. The amount of fortification can vary from food to food.

Almost any legume provides a nice amount of folate. One-half cup of lentils, for example, contains a hefty 179 micrograms of the nutrient. In the produce aisle and the frozen food section, check out asparagus, broccoli, okra, and spinach.

Vitamin B_6: All Systems Go

It may not have the name recognition of nutritional big guns like beta-carotene, calcium, and vitamin C. Yet vitamin B_6 performs a number of essential tasks within your body.

B_6 stands out as a major player in keeping your immune system strong. It helps transform food into energy and assists in the creation of neurotransmitters, the chemicals that enable brain cells to communicate with one another.

The list of conditions for which vitamin B_6 is gaining acceptance as a possible treatment continues to grow. Preliminary research suggests that it has the potential to protect against atherosclerosis and ease premenstrual symptoms. It also appears to improve your chances of conception.

Scientists cannot yet explain why, but B_6 also has the ability to stop the chronic wrist pain that characterizes carpal tunnel syndrome.

How much you need: The RDA of vitamin B_6 for women is 1.6 milligrams; the DV is 2 milligrams. That's not a whole lot, yet most women's diets come up short. For the therapeutic effects of the nutrient to kick in, you'd have to go even higher-perhaps as high as 10 milligrams, according to experts.

Where to get it: Almost any kind of fish can beef up your B$_6$ intake. For example, a 3-ounce serving of Atlantic mackerel supplies 0.4 milligram of the nutrient, or 20 percent of the DV. And rainbow trout supplies 17 percent of the DV. Or have a banana: One 4-ounce fruit gives you 0.7 milligram of B$_6$.

Vitamin C: A Most Prolific Protector

Call vitamin C the can-do nutrient. No other vitamin or mineral possesses C's ability to defend your body against an astounding array of illnesses, from the common cold to breast cancer.

Like beta-carotene and vitamin E, vitamin C is an antioxidant. It works by defusing those molecular time bombs known as free radicals, paving the way to good health. In studies of the relationship between vitamin C and cholesterol, for example, scientists have found that people with high levels of vitamin C in their blood have less chance of developing heart disease. In particular, women with high levels of vitamin C also have high levels of HDL cholesterol, the good kind that helps to keep your arteries clean.

Further, when researchers in Spain compared women who had breast cancer with women who didn't, they discovered that the breast cancer patients consumed fewer vitamin C–rich foods—namely, fruits and vegetables—in their diets.

There's evidence that vitamin C may even play a vital role in your body's bone-building process. When scientists examined the bone densities and eating habits of 775 postmenopausal women, they found that those with the sturdiest skeletons were getting daily doses of vitamin C along with their calcium. Even more noteworthy, for every 100 milligrams of C that these women ate, their bone densities were almost 2 percent higher, compared with the women who ate less vitamin C. Two percent may not sound like much, but every bit of bone that's spared puts one more step between you and the debilitation that osteoporosis can bring.

That's not all. Other research has linked vitamin C to a lower risk of chronic pulmonary disease—an umbrella term for respiratory diseases such as asthma, bronchitis, and emphysema—and to dramatically reduced progression of arthritis. The nutrient may also help protect the eyes, nerves, and kidneys from diabetes-related damage.

As for colds . . . well, contrary to popular belief, vitamin C can't stop you from getting one. But if you do get one, vitamin C has been proven to help chase it away. Pump yourself with vitamin C, and you can help make sure that your cold doesn't hang around for long and that its symptoms are less severe.

How much you need: When it comes to vitamin C, the experts say, "Fill 'er up!" Most recommend consuming 100 to 500 milligrams of the nutrient a day—roughly 1½ to 8 times the RDA for women, which is 60 milligrams.

Where to get it: Oranges are practically synonymous with vitamin C. Indeed, just one 4½-ounce fruit contains 70 milligrams of the nutrient—well above the RDA. But why not treat your tastebuds to other superior sources? Check out guava (165 milligrams), kiwifruit (75 milligrams), papaya (94 milligrams), and strawberries (85 milligrams), as well as broccoli (58 milligrams) and sweet red peppers (95 milligrams).

Vitamin E: Eat to Your Heart's Content

Like its antioxidant amigos vitamin C and beta-carotene, vitamin E neutralizes those disease-provoking free radicals that are floating around your system. The nutrient appears to play a prominent role in protecting you against the dastardly duo of heart disease and cancer.

Indeed, compelling research has reinforced the link between a high vitamin E intake and a healthy heart. Postmenopausal women who got lots of vitamin E from foods such as nuts and margarine had half the risk of a fatal heart attack over a period of 7 years, compared with women who consumed only small amounts.

Meanwhile, a study involving more than 600 women suggests that vitamin E may protect against cancer. The most dramatic protective effects occurred in women with family histories of breast cancer. Those who got the most vitamin E from foods managed to cut their chances of developing the disease by an impressive 80 percent, compared with other women. And among the women without family histories of breast cancer, consuming lots of vitamin E–rich foods produced a 40 percent dip in risk. The association between high vitamin E intake and reduced risk of breast cancer appeared strongest in premenopausal women.

There's also evidence that E can fend off respiratory problems and bolster your immune system's ability to combat infectious diseases.

How much you need: The "high-intake" women in the breast cancer study were getting roughly 10 IU of the nutrient a day—less than the RDA of 12 IU (8 milligrams alpha-tocopherol equivalents). Still, to get the most benefit from vitamin E, your daily intake should hover between 100 and 400 IU, experts advise. This exceeds even the DV of 30 IU.

Where to get it: The bad news about vitamin E

is that it's found primarily in high-fat vegetable oils and nuts. The good news is that you may not need all that much to experience its protective effects. For example, the women in the heart study with high intakes of vitamin E were actually eating only a few servings of nuts and margarine over the course of a week. Likewise, the high-intake women in the breast cancer study were getting less than the RDA.

Use high-fat vitamin E sources sparingly. Among oils, choose olive and peanut. Both have decent amounts of E, and most of their fat is the heart-healthy unsaturated kind. Wheat germ is also a good source: One-quarter cup, toasted, supplies roughly 40 percent of the RDA. Try sprinkling it on nonfat frozen yogurt and adding it to casseroles and baked goods.

Zinc: Don't "Cell" Yourself Short

Zinc specializes in cell production. When your body needs new cells—for healing, growth, or pregnancy—zinc works overtime to keep up with demand, according to Dr. Sherman.

Suppose, for example, you've been infected with a virus. Zinc joins forces with compounds called zinc-dependent enzymes to build new immune system cells to fight the infection.

Zinc's ability to replicate quickly comes in handy when you have a cut or wound. The mineral supports the production of collagen, the connective tissue that helps such injuries heal.

Zinc may also help to counteract the stay-away-from-me feelings that often accompany premenstrual syndrome. At least one study has found that zinc levels drop around the time of the month that premenstrual symptoms set in. This has led researchers to speculate that running low on the nutrient can unbalance the emotions, leading to mood swings.

How much you need: The RDA of zinc for women is 12 milligrams; the DV is 15 milligrams. Next to calcium, zinc is the mineral most often lacking in women's diets.

Where to get it: Just six medium steamed oysters provide 76 milligrams of zinc—a whopping 500 percent of the RDA. Lean meats and poultry are also excellent sources. Some whole-grain breads, cereals, and pasta contain decent amounts, as does nonfat yogurt.

The *Prevention* Food Pyramid for Women

What You Need Every Day

You may be a little rusty on the state capitals and the difference between an isosceles and an equilateral triangle. But we'd wager that at least one bit of grade school learning remains indelibly imprinted on your memory: the Four Food Groups.

Those were the days when meat was the main attraction in almost every meal, and veggies and fruits made only cameo appearances at the dinner table. That all changed in the early 1990s, when the U.S. Department of Agriculture officially concluded that the Basic Four no longer served the nutrition needs of the general population. They went back to the drawing board to come up with new, more realistic standards for what people should be eating.

Their efforts led to the creation of the Food Guide Pyramid, which has changed the way many of us look at our dinner plates. Grains, fruits, and vegetables have been given top priority, since they offer the most nutrients for the least amount of fat. Meats and dairy products, meanwhile, have been downsized from mainstays to virtual blips.

The Food Guide Pyramid is built on reams of scientific research into what constitutes a healthy diet. The question is, for whom?

Taking It Personally

"The Food Guide Pyramid purposely presents a very broad view of good nutrition so that it applies to the general population," says Joanne Curran-Celentano, R.D., Ph.D., associate professor of nutritional sciences at the University of New Hampshire in Durham. But in trying to be all things to all people, she explains, the pyramid ends up overlooking some very specific—and very important—nutrition needs among women.

For example, each food group in the pyramid lists a range of servings—a generous 6 to 11 for the grains that make up the pyramid's base. The low number applies to someone who requires just 1,600 calories a day, most likely a sedentary woman. The high number, on the other hand, is for someone who eats 2,800 calories a day, most likely an active man. How do you know where you fit in?

The pyramid also doesn't explain which foods supply the vitamins and minerals that women need most. "If you don't know of any other sources of calcium besides dairy products, for instance, you can take in way too many calories trying to meet the recommended daily intake of 1,000 milligrams," Dr. Curran-Celentano explains.

"There's no question that the Food Guide Pyramid is an improvement over the Four Food Groups and that it points us in the right direction for nutritional health," she adds. "But I think for it to be really useful for women, it should be redesigned with their specific nutrition needs in mind."

Making a Good Thing Better

Okay, we confess: We were hoping she'd say that. We, too, feel that it's about time for women-specific nutrition guidelines. So in collaboration with Dr. Curran-Celentano, we've created the first-ever *Prevention* Food Pyramid for Women.

The shape is familiar, but we've made some very important changes that can help you eat better and smarter. Use the pyramid as a guide in making your daily food choices to be sure you're getting the necessary mix of nutrients and the right number of calories to maintain a healthy weight. And you don't have to worry about counting grams of fat because the right amount is built into the serving sizes and numbers.

The Food Pyramid for Women is based on 1,800 calories a day. Compared with the original Food Guide Pyramid, this figure more closely aligns with what the typical moderately active woman between the ages of 35 and 50 consumes, Dr. Curran-Celentano explains.

Tied into the number of calories is what Dr. Curran-Celentano calls nutrient density. Women have to get more vitamins and minerals in fewer calories than men. This means that the foods you choose must supply lots of nutrients. So in the fruit and vegetable group, we've broken out the essentials—such as calcium, folate, and the carotenoids—and listed some of their best food sources.

Above all, the pyramid stresses variety, which Dr. Curran-Celentano feels is absolutely necessary for meeting all your nutrition needs. "There are women who say, 'I really like orange juice, so I'll just drink that to cover my fruit and vegetable servings for the day,'" she explains. "You may be getting enough servings, but you're not getting the mix of nutrients that other fruits and vegetables can provide." Besides, she adds, variety makes healthy eating interesting and fun.

"In a way, the pyramid is emancipating," Dr. Curran-Celentano says. "It lets you see that filling your meals with good, wholesome foods is actually very easy to do. And it gives you lots of choices, so you can have what you like." When you compare your current eating habits with the pyramid's recommendations, you may very well discover that you're not doing so badly after all. And if you are coming up short on certain key nutrients, consuming more of the right foods may be enough to put you over the top.

Navigating the Pyramid

The Food Pyramid for Women is tailored to accommodate a woman's specific nutrition needs. You can customize it even further, based on your calorie intake.

You may need more or less than the typical

woman's 1,800 calories per day, depending on your lifestyle and other factors. An active woman may require as many as 2,200 calories a day to fuel her body properly. Someone who's sedentary or trying to lose weight can make do with 1,600.

Those mathematical formulas you find in your doctor's office can help you figure out what your calorie intake should be, but they don't account for individual factors, such as your basal metabolism, that influence how many calories your body requires. A better method is to simply go by what feels right and comfortable to you.

For this plan to work, of course, you must be attuned to your appetite and your eating pattern. "Often women don't pay attention to their food choices and portion sizes, so they underestimate how much they're eating," Dr. Curran-Celentano explains. "They look at the pyramid and think, 'Wow! That's a lot of food!' But in reality, it's probably less than they're eating now. It's just spread out to include more types of foods, and the variety is more health-supporting."

Once you know your ideal calorie intake, you can pick and choose foods from each tier of the pyramid, using the serving numbers as guides in planning your daily menus. Remember, if you eat the recommended number of servings from each food group, you'll get just the right mix of nutrients that your body requires for good health.

Of course, many foods are good sources of not one but several nutrients. Such foods should serve single duty in your diet—in other words, select a different food from each category in the pyramid, suggests Dr. Curran-Celentano. Orange juice, for instance, supplies vitamin C and folate and may be calcium-fortified as well. So if orange juice is your folate source for the day,

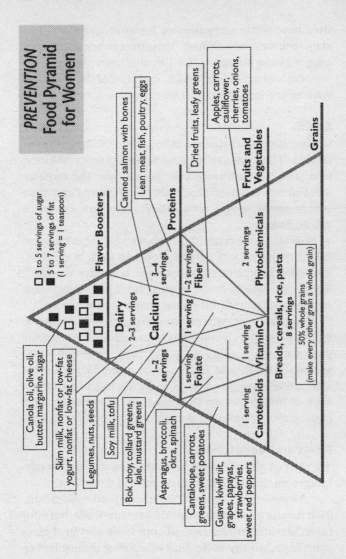

PREVENTION
Food Pyramid
for Women

☐ 3 to 5 servings of sugar
■ 5 to 7 servings of fat
(1 serving = 1 teaspoon)

Flavor Boosters

Canola oil, olive oil, butter, margarine, sugar

Dairy
2–3 servings

Skim milk, nonfat or low-fat yogurt, nonfat or low-fat cheese

Calcium
3–4 servings

Canned salmon with bones

Proteins

Lean meat, fish, poultry, eggs

1–2 servings

Legumes, nuts, seeds

Soy milk, tofu

Bok choy, collard greens, kale, mustard greens

Fiber
1–2 servings

Dried fruits, leafy greens

Fruits and Vegetables

Apples, carrots, cauliflower, cherries, onions, tomatoes

Phytochemicals
2 servings

Folate
1 serving

Asparagus, broccoli, okra, spinach

Vitamin C
1 serving

Carotenoids
1 serving

Cantaloupe, carrots, greens, sweet potatoes

Guava, kiwifruit, grapes, papayas, strawberries, sweet red peppers

Breads, cereals, rice, pasta
8 servings

50% whole grains
(make every other grain a whole grain)

Grains

43

then have some strawberries for your vitamin C and skim milk for your calcium. This strategy boosts your intake of all the nutrients, Dr. Curran-Celentano says.

Let's take a closer look at each tier of the pyramid, starting at the bottom and working our way up.

Grains

Grains supply carbohydrates, your body's fuel of choice. They also offer generous amounts of fiber, iron, and B vitamins. Whole grains have the most to offer, nutrition-wise. That's why Dr. Curran-Celentano recommends that every other grain you eat be a whole grain.

What about pasta? "I think we've gone a bit overboard with it," Dr. Curran-Celentano says. "Certainly, it's a good source of carbohydrates, but that's about it." There are whole-grain pastas available, which are better than the refined pastas that most people eat.

Servings: If you're following an 1,800-calorie eating plan, Dr. Curran-Celentano advises aiming for eight servings of grains a day. Women consuming 1,600 calories a day should go for six servings; 2,200 calories a day, nine servings. A serving equals half of a bagel, a slice of bread, ¾ cup dry, ready-to-eat cereal, ½ cup cooked rice or pasta, or 3 cups of air-popped popcorn.

Fruits and Vegetables

This tier of the pyramid actually consists of five subgroups, each one featuring an essential nutrient.

Vitamin C. Vitamin C from food is an antioxidant. That means it helps to neutralize free radicals, harmful molecules that travel around your body and steal electrons from healthy molecules to stabilize themselves (a process known as oxidation). By incapacitating free radicals, vitamin C helps protect against serious health problems, including heart disease and cancer.

Servings: Everyone—regardless of calorie intake—should try to consume at least one serving of a vitamin C–rich food a day, Dr. Curran-Celentano says. A serving can be ½ cup of broccoli, strawberries, or sweet peppers, or a 6-ounce glass of orange, grapefruit, or tomato juice.

Folate. "This B vitamin has really come into its own in recent years," Dr. Curran-Celentano says. "Before we just thought of it in terms of keeping red blood cells healthy. But now we know it can do much more than that." It helps protect developing fetuses from neural tube defects, serious complications that affect the brain and spine. And it appears to lower a woman's risk of heart disease.

Servings: No matter what your calorie intake, Dr. Curran-Celentano suggests that you try for at least one serving of a folate-rich food a day. Suggestions include a 6-ounce glass of orange juice, ½ cup of cooked asparagus or broccoli, or 1 cup of raw spinach.

Phytochemicals. These little-known compounds may turn out to be our most potent weapons against disease, if the latest research is any indication. The catch is that you can get them only from fruits, vegetables, and other plant sources—at least for now. So squeeze some phyto-rich foods into your daily menu.

Servings: Dr. Curran-Celentano recommends at least two servings of top-notch phytochemical sources a day for everyone, regardless of calorie intake. Among the best: ½ cup of tomatoes, ½ cup of cooked broccoli, and ½ cup of kale.

Carotenoids. Beta-carotene is probably the best known of the carotenoid clan. Your body converts many of these compounds—which are, incidentally, phytochemicals—to vitamin A, a nutrient that's essential for normal vision and a strong immune system. But the carotenoids are showing promise in their own right as potential protectors against heart disease and cancer.

Servings: One a day for everyone, Dr. Curran-Celentano says. Choose from 6 ounces of apricot nectar, one-quarter of a cantaloupe, or ½ cup of cooked carrots, sweet potatoes, or greens.

Fiber. Technically, fiber doesn't qualify as a nutrient, because it passes through your body without getting absorbed. What it does is add bulk to the foods that you eat, which helps you feel full on fewer calories while keeping your digestive system working smoothly. Fiber may also bind with cholesterol and bile acids and escort them out of your body.

Servings: Women who are consuming 1,800 calories a day should aim for one to two servings of fiber-rich fruits and vegetables a day, according to Dr. Curran-Celentano. Those following 1,600-calorie plans can get by with one serving, while those on the 2,200-calorie plan require at least two servings. Good choices include ¼ cup of dried fruit, 1 cup of a leafy green, and ½ cup of any other vegetable.

Proteins

Your body uses protein to carry out a variety of tasks. It helps to build and maintain all of your muscles—including your heart muscle—and supports the production of hormones, blood cells, and immune cells. You should get half of your protein from animal sources and the other half from legumes and soy foods. Of course, if you're a vegetarian, you can get all of your protein from plant sources.

Dairy. In addition to protein, dairy products

such as milk, cheese, and yogurt supply generous amounts of calcium, your body's premier bone-builder. Fortified milk may be your skeleton's best friend. It delivers calcium as well as vitamin D, which your body needs in order to absorb the mineral.

Servings: All women should consume two to three servings of nonfat or low-fat dairy products a day, states Dr. Curran-Celentano. Help yourself to 8 ounces of skim milk, 1 cup of nonfat or low-fat yogurt, 1½ ounces of nonfat or low-fat cheese, or 2 ounces of processed cheese. If you are lactose-intolerant or you avoid dairy products for other reasons, you can substitute 1 cup of fortified soy milk or 2 ounces of soy cheese, both of which are good sources of calcium.

Meats. Think of it as meats-plus: This protein category also includes poultry, fish, legumes, and soy products. Many of these foods supply healthy doses of iron and zinc, two essential nutrients that women routinely run low on. Iron, in particular, can be a problem for some women because the body's stores of the mineral are depleted every month during menstruation.

Soy is shaping up to be a real nutrition superstar, according to Dr. Curran-Celentano. Studies suggest that it may help to lower cholesterol and to boost bone density. It's also rich in phytoestrogens, phytochemicals that have the potential to protect against breast cancer. "I'd certainly recommend trying to eat soy foods at least several times a week," Dr. Curran-Celentano says.

Servings: Dr. Curran-Celentano recommends that all women consume up to six servings of these protein-rich foods every day. Of that number, one to two servings should come from nonmeat sources. One ounce of lean beef, chicken, or fish constitutes a serving, as does one egg, ½ cup of legumes, 2 table-

spoons of peanut butter, or 1 ounce of tofu. By combining meat and nonmeat sources, you get more variety in your diet over the course of the day. That
makes it easier to meet your body's nutrient needs.

Calcium
We've already mentioned that milk and other dairy
products are top-notch sources of calcium. The fact is,
you can get the mineral from a variety of foods, including fish, soy products, and produce. That explains
why calcium holds the place of honor at the center of
the pyramid, overlapping all three tiers. Your body
uses the mineral for many tasks besides bone-building,
including muscle function and heartbeat regulation.
But the bottom line is that stocking up on calcium
now can spare you the debilitating effects of bone loss
later in life, Dr. Curran-Celentano says.

Servings: All women should eat at least one
serving of a calcium-rich vegetable a day in addition to
the two to three servings of dairy foods (or soy-based
substitutes) mentioned earlier, recommends Dr.
Curran-Celentano. So help yourself to ½ cup of broccoli, or a dark, leafy green such as kale or bok choy.
Other excellent nondairy sources of calcium include 3
ounces of canned salmon with bones, 3 ounces of
tofu, 6 ounces of fortified soy milk, and 6 ounces of
calcium-fortified orange juice.

Flavor Boosters
The Food Pyramid for Women allows for moderate
amounts of fat and sugar—what Dr. Curran-Celentano
refers to as flavor boosters. You'll find them at the very
top of the pyramid. Both have their place in good nutrition: Sugar is a carbohydrate, while fats such as veg-

etable oils supply vitamin E, an antioxidant that preliminary research has linked to a reduced risk of heart disease. Including them in the pyramid also serves an important psychological purpose. "It's expected that you're going to eat a chocolate chip cookie once in a while, so the pyramid is designed to accommodate that," Dr. Curran-Celentano explains. "It's all part of eating healthfully." Still, she says, you don't want to add seven pats of butter to one food item and use up all your flavor boosters in one sitting. Spread them out all through the day.

Servings: If you're following an 1,800-calorie eating plan, you can have five to seven servings of fat per day, according to Dr. Curran-Celentano. A serving equals 1 teaspoon of a vegetable oil (preferably olive or canola oil) or 1 teaspoon of butter or margarine. As for sugar, the pyramid allows for three to five servings a day, with a serving being the equivalent of 1 teaspoon.

How does this work? Well, suppose you have reduced-fat milk rather than skim on your breakfast cereal. That means you should skip the pat of butter on your dinner roll.

Key Nutrients for Men

Better Living through Chemistry

Men and women are different.

That's something that sounds obvious, but what we're talking about here are subtle nutritional differences. Yes, like the average woman, you probably could stand to reduce the amount of fat in your diet, increase carbohydrates, eat more fiber, and eat foods that are rich in vitamins and minerals. But when it comes to the specific foods you need—and how much of them you should eat—you, as a man, set a course of your own.

Examples:

♦ *Calories.* Just to maintain your body you need to get about 1,000 calories more per day than the average woman.

♦ *Minerals.* Women need to get 15 milligrams of iron a day; if you took that much it could increase your risk of heart disease.

♦ *Vitamins.* In some cases, like vitamin C, you and the average woman need the same amount. In other cases (B_6 is one) it takes 20 percent more to fill your tank.

Obviously, when it comes to nutrition this isn't a one-size-fits-all world. In this chapter, we'll look at your specific needs and explain the best ways to meet them, as well as some ways you should avoid.

Carbohydrates: Power to the People

Your body can burn a number of substances for energy—fat, protein, and even alcohol. But your body doesn't suffer these fuels gladly. Eating a lot of fat can lead to nasty diseases, like cancer and heart disease. When your body has to rely on protein for energy, it's not satisfied with the meat and eggs you eat—it starts dismantling your muscle tissue, too. And alcohol is a nutritional bully: Not only does it feed you "empty" calories, meaning you get zip for sustenance, but it also wreaks havoc with your liver, your brain, and the nutritional metabolism in your bodily tissues.

So it's no wonder that you hear so much glowing praise for carbohydrates. They're a top-notch energy source, and the foods that tend to provide them—fruits, vegetables, beans, and grains—are low in fat and high in fiber.

"There is a strong drive toward reducing fat intake, and the only way to do that and to maintain an adequate amount of caloric intake is to increase the consumption of carbohydrates," says Benjamin Caballero, M.D., Ph.D., director of the Center for Human Nutrition at Johns Hopkins University in Baltimore.

The typical male between ages 20 and 50 gets about 47 percent of his calories from carbohydrates. Americans were getting 56 percent in the early 1900s. The proportion of complex carbohydrates in the American diet, however, has plunged by more

Carbohydrate Sources

Here is the carbohydrate content in grams of commonly consumed foods.

Food	Grams of Carbohydrates
Apple	21
Baked potato	21
Banana	26
Bran flakes, 1 oz	25
Bread, white, 1 slice	15
Bread, whole-wheat, 1 slice	13
Cheese, Cheddar, 1 oz	7.2
Corn, canned, 4 oz	19.8
Cornflakes, 1 oz	25
Green beans, 4 oz	10
Hamburger, 3 oz	0
Milk, 2%, 8 oz	5
Milk, whole, 8 oz	4.7
Peach	10
Peanut butter, 2 Tbsp	5.4
Rice, 1 oz	24
Saltine crackers, 4	7
Shredded Wheat, 1 biscuit	26
Tomato	5.3

than 30 percent since the turn of the century, while consumption of sugar, a simple carbohydrate, has soared. Nutrition experts recommend men get 55 to 60 percent of their total calories from carbohydrates, and that no more than 10 percent be from added sugar.

Proteins: The Original Bodybuilders

If proteins were people, they'd all have answering machines, car phones, and chock-full appointment calendars. They are busy little chains of amino acids.

Your body is constantly tearing down and building up tissues, which means it has to destroy and then recreate proteins perpetually. Every 4 to 6 days, for instance, you get an entirely new intestinal wall.

Pick a reaction in the body, and there's probably a protein enzyme behind it. Proteins carry oxygen in your blood. They slide against each other to make your muscles contract. As photoreceptors, they suck up light for your vision.

"Proteins are the building blocks of practically everything in our bodies," says Dr. Caballero. "Particularly, the skeletal muscle and all of the organs that make us function are made of protein."

Not sure you're getting enough protein? Most likely, you have no need to worry. A survey of more than 50,000 people showed that American men commonly consume as much as 110 grams of protein a day—far more than necessary. Only 2 percent of the American population was getting less than 80 percent of the recommended amount.

"The American diet has excessive protein," says Dr. Caballero. "The human body doesn't have any way to store protein, so if you eat a lot of protein, you are going to eliminate it in the urine. It's not clear whether that's detrimental to health in the long term, but certainly it makes your kidneys work more, because the kidneys have to get rid of all that extra protein."

An international panel of nutrition experts recommends that men should eat at least one-third of a gram of protein for every pound of body weight each day. If you weigh 165 pounds, for example, your safe minimum is about 56 grams of protein. Their recommended level at that weight is slightly higher: 62 grams a day.

Where's the Protein?

Here is the protein content in grams for a typical serving of common foods.

Food	Grams of Protein
Apple	0.3
Bacon, 3 slices	6
Baked potato	3
Banana	1.1
Bread, white, 1 slice	2
Bread, whole-wheat, 1 slice	3
Cheese, Cheddar, 1 oz	7
Chicken, 3 oz	27
Corn, canned, 4 oz	2.5
Cornflakes, 1 cup	2

Vitamins: The Chemical Alphabet Soup

Vitamins are the diplomatic corps of the body. With a quiet nudge here and a gentle stroke there, their minuscule ranks wield a huge influence over the processes of your body. It's also a sure bet we don't know everything they're up to.

What we do know is that vitamins are substances the body needs in tiny amounts before a host of chemical processes can happen, particularly interactions with enzymes and the release of energy from carbo-

Food	Grams of Protein
Egg, fried, 1 large	6
Green beans, 4 oz	1
Green peas, 4 oz	4
Hamburger, 3 oz	21
Kidney beans, ½ cup	7.5
Milk, whole or 2%, 8 oz	8
Peanut butter, 2 Tbsp	10
Pork, 3 oz	23
Rice, ½ cup cooked	2
Roast beef, 3 oz	19
Shredded Wheat, 1 biscuit	3
Tomato	1
Tuna, 3 oz	24

hydrates, protein, and fat. They play many other roles, aiding in such things as vision, hormone production, and immunity.

Some vitamins also help protect you from the leading men-killer diseases. Beta-carotene (a form of vitamin A) and vitamins C and E have gained a lot of attention for their antioxidant qualities. This means they may counteract the free radicals in your body that are linked to cancer and cardiovascular disease.

The Best Source: Food

Nutrition experts say the very best way to get your vitamins is to eat lots of different, wholesome foods—particularly fruits and vegetables. A vitamin pill will supply you with important, but narrowly specified, chemicals. Real food covers the nutritional bases much more thoroughly, not only with vitamins and minerals but also with carbohydrates, protein, fiber, and, probably, some crucial substances that haven't even been identified yet.

"I would recommend trying to consume at least five servings of vegetables and fresh fruits every day. There is clear evidence that people who do that have less incidence of a number of diseases," says Dr. Caballero. "There are hundreds of substances we don't know anything about in fruits and vegetables, and a lot of them have antioxidant properties. It is still uncertain which group of them is actually active."

In special circumstances, your diet may fall short of what you need to stay healthy, and you should huddle with your doctor about whether you need a boost from supplements. Maybe you've been dieting long-term, have food allergies, take certain medications, drink alcohol excessively, or follow a vegetarian diet. And maybe, despite your best efforts, you've spent too much time in the shadow of the golden arches and you'd like some nutritional insurance.

If supplements are appropriate for you, you should pick one carefully. Here are guidelines from Dr. Liz Applegate of *Runner's World* magazine.

Get the right balance. Find a supplement that provides 100 to 150 percent of the Daily Value for the 13 recognized vitamins, plus zinc, selenium, and, if possible, copper. It also should contain smaller amounts of iron, calcium, and magnesium. Men require less iron than women, and an excess may be linked to heart disease because it's a powerful oxidant. So make sure the iron content is at or below 10 milligrams. Calcium and magnesium should be present at 10 to 25 percent of their Daily Values. The Daily Value for calcium is 1,000 milligrams; for magnesium it is 400 milligrams.

Save your dough. Pass on a supplement that requires you to take three or four doses a day. That's an expensive hassle. Generic brands are generally just as good as the costlier stuff. Time-release pills and effervescence are expensive gimmicks, and natural or organic sources for vitamins aren't necessarily better, explains Dr. Applegate.

Pass on the extras. Supplements labeled "high potency" or "therapeutic" typically contain excessive doses that may be hazardous. Forgo such nonessential, unproven nutrients as rose hips, "vitamin B$_{15}$," inositol, PABA, rutin, and bioflavonoids, Dr. Applegate says.

Forget megadosing. Many vitamins and minerals become toxic and even deadly in large doses, so a more-is-better philosophy is foolhardy. At the very least you're flushing gold down the toilet, literally and figuratively, since the excess of many vitamins comes out in your urine. But fat-soluble vitamins, like A, D, and E, can build up dangerously in your body, Dr. Applegate says. Moderation, then, is the best policy. Here are the vitamins you need in your diet and their recommended amounts.

Vitamin A

Role: Required for normal vision, reproduction, cell development, growth, and immunity. Beta-carotene, chemically related to vitamin A, is an antioxidant.

Major sources: Liver, egg yolks, whole-milk products, cantaloupes, peaches, carrots, cooked spinach, broccoli, tomatoes, lettuce, green peas, green beans, and canned corn.

How much men need: The Daily Value is 5,000 international units (IU) (1,000 micrograms RE—retinol equivalents), what you would get by consuming 3 ounces of tuna, one 8-ounce glass of whole milk, 2 ounces of Cheddar cheese, or ½ cup of cooked spinach.

Vitamin D

Role: Aids absorption of calcium, bone-building and nerve-muscle interaction.

Major sources: Canned sardines, canned salmon, canned herring, and fortified foods, like milk.

How much men need: The Daily Value is 400 IU (10 micrograms), what you would get in a quart of fortified milk.

Vitamin E

Role: This antioxidant protects a wide range of chemicals, cells, and tissues from oxidation damage.

Major sources: Superfortified cereals (containing added vitamins and minerals), shellfish, greens (mustard, turnip, kale, collards), fried fish, fried potatoes, spaghetti with tomato sauce, chili, peanuts, peanut butter, chicken dishes, and pizza.

How much men need: The Daily Value is 30 IU (20 milligrams α–TE—alpha-tocopherol equivalents), the amount you would get by eating a serving of spaghetti with tomato sauce, coleslaw, greens, fried potatoes, and a slice of pie.

Vitamin K

Role: Helps to regulate clotting in the blood.

Major sources: Green leafy vegetables, fruits, tubers, seeds, eggs, dairy products, and meats.

How much men need: No Daily Value recommended. The RDA is 80 micrograms (about four spears of broccoli).

Vitamin C

Role: Necessary in the bone-building process, the formation of neurotransmitters, the activation of hormones, and detoxification processes in the liver. It helps the body use iron, calcium, and folic acid. Vitamin C also is an important antioxidant.

Major sources: Oranges, grapefruits, cantaloupes, sweet red peppers, raw spinach, steamed broccoli, and fortified cereals.

How much men need: The Daily Value is 60 milligrams, which you would get in a single orange. Optimal dosage is much debated, however, and some researchers advise anywhere from 250 to 1,000 milligrams a day.

Folic Acid

Role: Required for the growth and division of the cells of all life forms. Fast-growing cells, such as red blood cells, are particularly sensitive to deficiencies.

Major sources: Liver; cold cereals; pinto, navy, and other dried beans; spinach; asparagus; seeds; okra; and broccoli.

How much men need: The Daily Value is 0.4 milligram (400 micrograms), the amount that you would get by eating one serving of regular cold cereal and a serving each of pinto or navy beans, broccoli, and okra.

Cobalamin (B_{12})

Role: Essential for DNA synthesis and cell division. Red blood cell production is particularly sensitive to deficiencies.

Major sources: Liver, oysters, roast beef, ground beef, bacon, ham, whole milk, and fried eggs.

How much men need: The Daily Value is 6 micrograms, which you would get by consuming 6 ounces of tuna and two 8-ounce glasses of whole milk.

Pyridoxine (B_6)

Role: Involved in nearly all aspects of protein and amino acid metabolism.

Major sources: Chicken, fish, whole-grain cereals, egg yolks, bananas, avocados, and potatoes.

How much men need: The more protein in the diet, the more vitamin B_6 you need. The Daily Value is 2 milligrams, which you would get by eating a chicken breast, a baked potato, and a cup of navy beans.

Thiamin

Role: Involved in the metabolism of carbohydrates.

Major sources: Pork, peas, beans, whole grains, and fortified breads.

How much men need: The Daily Value is 1.5 milligrams, which you would get from one serving each of cornflakes, orange juice , ham, peas, rice, baked potato, and whole-wheat bread.

Riboflavin

Role: Involved in growth and repair of tissues; release of energy from blood sugar, fatty acids, and amino acids; production of hormones; and formation of red blood cells.

Major sources: Milk, liver, kidney, whole grains, fortified breads, broccoli, asparagus, potatoes, peas, and orange juice.

How much men need: The Daily Value is 1.7 milligrams, which you would get by having one serving each of cornflakes, roast beef, milk, low-fat cottage cheese, broccoli, and a banana.

Niacin

Role: Essential for the release of energy from carbohydrates, fat, protein, and alcohol.

Major sources: Baked goods, cereals, meats, tea, coffee, and beer.

How much men need: The Daily Value is 20 milligrams (20 milligrams NE—niacin equivalents), which you would get by consuming one serving each of cornflakes, chicken, whole-wheat bread, and canned corn.

Pantothenic Acid (B₅)

Role: Aids in the metabolism of carbohydrates, fat, and protein and helps to synthesize hormones, neurotransmitters, and other essential compounds.

Major sources: Raw avocados, raw broccoli, bran, organ meats, dry milk, and eggs.

How much men need: The Daily Value is 10 milligrams. You could get that by eating two servings each of liver, broccoli, avocados, and brown rice.

Biotin

Role: Biotin has a variety of metabolic roles, including the synthesis and oxidation of fatty acids, oxidation of carbohydrates, and the metabolizing of several amino acids. It also helps the immune system function.

Major sources: Liver, kidney, peanut butter, egg yolks, yeast, cauliflower, legumes, nuts, and cereals.

How much men need: The Daily Value is 0.3 milligram (300 micrograms). You would get that by consuming one serving each of liver, green beans, nuts, and oatmeal.

Minerals: The Basic Dirt

Name a bodily process and there's bound to be a mineral involved. Enzymes are behind virtually every chemical reaction in your body, and a third of the known enzymes need mineral ions around before they can do their thing. Non-enzyme proteins make use of minerals, too. Hemoglobin, for example, uses iron ions to bind itself to oxygen, which is carted around your bloodstream by hemoglobin.

While they're crucial to life, the minerals in your body don't amount to much bulk. Pile together all 56 of the minerals known to be in a 165-pound man, and you'd have just enough dirt for a couple of mud pies— less than 7 pounds.

Scientists say 16 of those minerals—including the ones detailed below—are essential, meaning you couldn't live, grow, or reproduce without them. Eleven others, including silicon, nickel, fluoride, and tin, are involved somehow in biological reactions.

Mining for Good Health

While Americans typically get an adequate balance of minerals in their food, two minerals are particularly worth keeping an eye on, says Dr. Caballero. "Zinc is linked to spermatogenesis—it's important for development of the gonads," he says. "Although the usual diet can provide the correct amount, this is a nutrient you need to make sure you get enough of. The main source of zinc in the diet is animal meat.

"The other mineral to consider for men is iron. In women, the risk with iron is deficiency. In men, it is the opposite. There already are two or three major studies showing that the more iron men have in their blood the more risk they have of heart disease." Iron is thought to oxidize fat in the bloodstream, he says, causing it to cling to artery walls, which leads to arteriosclerosis.

Men should avoid taking iron supplements unless they are taking them under a doctor's supervision, for short periods of time, to treat anemia. It's not likely that you would get excess iron from food.

"The absorption of iron from the intestine is tightly regulated," Dr. Caballero says. "So it's unlikely that you could get too much iron, for example, by eating a lot of beef. It would have to be from taking a lot of supplements on a regular basis, at least for several months."

Here's a rundown of several minerals that are important to your health.

Zinc

Role: This mineral is important to your sex drive, fertility, wound healing, immunity, and the senses of smell and taste.

Major sources: Lean beef, turkey, oysters, cereal, beans, and wheat germ.

How much men need: The Daily Value is 15 milligrams, which you would get in a serving of roast beef, ½ cup of oysters, 1 cup of beans, and two 8-ounce glasses of whole milk.

Calcium

Role: Crucial for bone formation and prevention of osteoporosis, blood clotting, and neurotransmitter function. By the way, osteoporosis—bones weakened by a lack of calcium—is not just a women's disease. A third of the broken hips related to osteoporosis occur in men.

Major sources: Milk, cheese, yogurt, ice cream, sardines, almonds, sesame seeds, broccoli, green leafy vegetables, and soybeans.

How much men need: The Daily Value is 1,000 milligrams, which you would get in two 8-ounce glasses of skim milk and two servings of broccoli.

Copper

Role: Helps to prevent heart disease and assists T-cells and antibodies in the immune system.

Major sources: Liver, shellfish, nuts, cocoa, mushrooms, whole-grain cereals, gelatin, peas, beans, and fruits.

How much men need: The Daily Value is 2 milligrams a day. Three or four oysters would do it. So would 3 ounces of Alaskan king crab, a baked potato with the skin, and 1 cup of white beans.

Magnesium

Role: Crucial for muscle activity, conduction of nerve impulses, and protection against heart disease.

Major sources: Vegetables, legumes, seafood, nuts, and dairy products.

How much men need: The Daily Value is 400

milligrams, which you would get by eating 1 cup of spinach, two servings of broccoli, 1 ounce of sunflower seeds, and 2 tablespoons of peanut butter.

Selenium

Role: A component of certain proteins, selenium is particularly known for assisting antioxidant protection.

Major sources: Organ meats, meat, fish, cereals, dairy products, broccoli, cucumbers, onions, garlic, radishes, and mushrooms. The more protein in your food, the more selenium you get.

How much men need: No Daily Value. The RDA is 70 micrograms. Three ounces of canned tuna would put you over the top.

Iron

Role: Involved in the transportation of oxygen and formation of red blood cells.

Major sources: Liver, meat, fish, poultry, cereal products, apricots, kidney beans, potatoes, peas, raw spinach, and raw broccoli.

How much men need: The RDA is 10 milligrams. Three ounces of roast tenderloin, a cup of enriched raisin bran, and a baked potato (with the skin) would do the trick. But before you load up your plate, consider: Men hold on to their iron better than women and generally don't need extra. And remember, there's evidence that high iron stores can contribute to heart disease.

Fiber: Straight Talk

Fiber keeps your digestive system active and productive, and with that comes a number of important health benefits.

For example:

♦ A high-fiber diet helps to protect you from cancer of the colon, possibly because it sweeps carcinogens out of the intestines more quickly or because it encourages advantageous chemical reactions in the digestive tract.

♦ Fiber produces soft, bulky feces, preventing the inflammation that comes with harder stools. Researchers from Harvard University and Brigham and Women's Hospital in Boston tracked 48,000 men for 4 years and found that those who ate lots of fiber in the form of fruits and vegetables were 42 percent less likely to develop diverticular disease than those who got the least fiber in their diets.

♦ It helps to lower cholesterol, leaving you less prone to heart disease.

♦ While you're consuming foods high in fiber—fruits, vegetables, and whole grains—you're usually getting another dietary bonus: complex carbohydrates.

Nutrition experts recommend consuming 20 to 30 grams of fiber a day. Five daily servings of fruits and vegetables and six servings of grains (the less processing the better) will do the trick. American men typically get only 15 grams a day.

"In our country, where we consume a lot of processed food, fiber intake is extremely low," says Dr. Caballero. "Therefore, we have an effort by industry to add back the fiber and by people to consume more unprocessed foods."

Fiber In, Fiber Out

Fiber is indigestible carbohydrate. It sweeps all the way through your digestive system without being absorbed into the body. There are two kinds.

Fiber Options

Here is the dietary fiber content in grams of some common foods.

Food	Grams of Fiber
Apple	2.6
Baked potato	1.4
Banana	1.4
Bran flakes, 1 oz	8.2
Bread, white, 1 slice	0.8
Bread, whole-wheat, 1 slice	2.4
Corn, canned, 4 oz	1.3
Cornflakes, 1 oz	2.8
Green beans, 4 oz	1.8
Green peas, 4 oz	5.4
Hamburger, 3 oz	0
Peanut butter, 2 Tbsp	2.1
Shredded Wheat, 1 biscuit	3

♦ Insoluble fiber, such as cellulose. This does for your stool what it once did for that squash or carrot you ate: It gives it bulk.

♦ Soluble fiber, found in fruits, some legumes, and grains. This stuff forms a gel that slows the rate at which food passes through the small intestine, thus increasing the absorption of nutrients. It also increases the excretion of bile acids and slows the rate of cholesterol absorption. Some soluble fibers trap bile acids in the gut, according to one theory. The body makes bile acids out of cholesterol, so when soluble fiber escorts them out of the body, the liver has to pull cholesterol from the blood to make more. The result: lower cholesterol.

Dr. Caballero recommends that people increase their fiber intake just by eating the right foods. But if you're having trouble wolfing down that much plant food for some reason, the fiber supplements available in drugstores are a reasonable backup.

"You have to try the supplements and see which one fits," says Dr. Caballero. "Some of those fibers are produced by a fermented bacteria and may produce a lot of gas or even cramps. But there's nothing wrong with them."

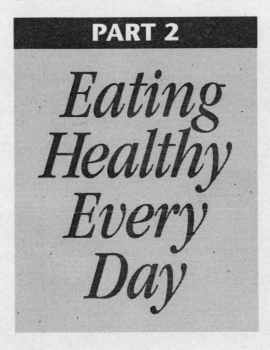

PART 2

*Eating
Healthy
Every
Day*

The Healthy Kitchen

Stocking Up Smart

Healthy cooking has long had a reputation as a time-consuming, costly, complicated venture. The truth is that it doesn't require exotic ingredients or expensive equipment. For that matter, it doesn't require any special culinary skills. Even a novice can prepare nutritious meals quickly and easily.

The real trick to healthy cooking, nutritionists agree, is to heed the Boy Scout motto "Be prepared." That means stocking up—filling your pantry and refrigerator with nutritious, versatile staples and outfitting your kitchen with quality, user-friendly gear. What you choose to have on hand really depends on your personal likes and dislikes as well as your lifestyle. And if you're feeding a family, you'll need to consider their preferences as well. The idea is to create an environment that encourages healthy cooking by putting all the essential supplies within reach.

First-Rate Fixin's

The following foods are recommended by nutritionists and chefs as healthy-cooking essentials. Consider this list a jumping-off point for stocking (or restocking) your own kitchen. As you try new recipes and develop healthier versions of old favorites, you'll come up with your own collection of can't-do-without ingredients. Keep in mind, too, that you don't necessarily want a lot of each item on hand. Buying in small quantities ensures that what you have is fresh.

Canned tomato puree. Tomatoes are brimming with lycopene, a nutritional newcomer that in studies appears to protect against cervical dysplasia as well as several different types of cancer. You can whip up a low-fat, nutrient-rich spaghetti sauce or pizza topping by blending tomato puree with garlic and spices. Just be sure the tomato product you choose is low in sodium.

Chili peppers. These potent peppers pack intense flavor, not to mention a healthy dose of vitamins A and C. "If you're not used to cooking with chili peppers, always remember to wear rubber gloves when cutting them," cautions award-winning chef Rick Bayless, author of *Rick Bayless's Mexican Kitchen*. "The oil contained in the membranes and the seed pods— not the seeds themselves—can irritate your skin."

Citrus fruits. The citric acid in oranges, lemons, limes, and grapefruit is a natural flavor enhancer that's especially adept at giving pizzazz to low-sodium dishes. Use the juices from these fruits liberally in everything from salad dressings and soups to stir-fries and desserts. They'll give you a burst of vitamin C to boot.

Grains. Quick-cooking varieties—including bulgur, couscous, millet, oats, and some types of barley and brown rice—can be ready in half an hour or less, so you can prepare them even when you're pressed for time. Cooked grains also freeze well.

Herbs and spices. No healthy kitchen should be without them! Use these seasonings instead of fat and salt when you cook. The flavor of fresh herbs is diminished with long cooking, so it's best to add them to a dish just before serving. Dried herbs benefit from longer cooking to rehydrate them and release their flavors.

Legumes. Beans, peas, and lentils can't be beat for fiber content. They're also good sources of protein, which makes them ideal substitutes for meat in all types of dishes. Dried beans do take a long time to cook, but you can use canned beans in most recipes. Just be sure to rinse them well to wash away the thick liquid—and some of the excess sodium—that they're packed in. Among the most versatile legumes are black beans, chickpeas, kidney beans, lentils, lima beans, pea beans, pinto beans, and split peas.

Onion-family vegetables. This odoriferous clan includes garlic, leeks, scallions, shallots, chives—and, of course, onions. Use them liberally to add flavor to savory dishes of all types. Cooking onions slowly gives them a sweet, mild taste. Leeks are inherently mild, as are Vidalia, Walla Walla, and Maui onions. Roasting garlic tames its sharp flavor and softens it to a creamy consistency. If you grow chives, let them flower, and then sprinkle the flower petals over salads.

Pasta. Pasta cooks up quickly for a fast low-fat meal. Look for enriched pasta, which supplies healthy doses of a number of vitamins and minerals, most notably niacin and thiamin, both B vitamins. But you can easily destroy pasta's natural goodness by drowning it in a fatty cream sauce. Be sure to stick with a lighter topping—for example, one made from fresh tomatoes. Read labels when buying pasta; many types of fresh pasta have considerably more fat and cholesterol than dried.

Tofu. This soy product is rich in phytoestrogens—supernutrients that have been shown to minimize the physical effects of menopause and to reduce the risk of breast cancer. Tofu is also an excellent source of protein, so you can use it instead of meat. It does taste bland when served plain, but it readily takes on flavors from other ingredients. Freezing tofu and then thawing and crumbling it gives it the texture of ground meat.

Tortillas. You can wrap just about any filling in this low-fat Mexican bread for a quick and easy lunch or dinner. Or top it with low-sodium tomato sauce or salsa, sliced vegetables, and shredded low-fat cheese for a personal pizza. Corn tortillas are your best nutritional choice. One 6-inch corn tortilla contains less than 0.5 gram of fat compared with over 2 grams for a 6-inch flour tortilla.

Gearing Up

Of course, no healthy kitchen is complete without some essential tools. The key word here is *essential*: It's not necessary to buy one of each gadget on display in the housewares section of your local department store. You can prepare just about any meal with a carefully selected collection of small appliances, cookware, and utensils.

To get you started, here's a list of equipment that nutritionists and healthy chefs consider must-haves in the kitchen. They make healthy cooking a breeze by helping to reduce the fat content of foods while preserving their nutrition and flavor.

Egg separator. For years, eggs have gotten a bad rap because of their high cholesterol content. The fact is that all that cholesterol is concentrated in the yolk. The white, on the other hand, has no cholesterol, no fat, and hardly any calories. It's also an excellent source of protein. An egg separator makes it easy to strain the white from the yolk without breaking the yolk.

Electric spice grinder. Freshly ground spices have much more intense, robust flavors than pre-ground varieties. An electric coffee grinder reserved for spices does the job in just seconds. It also comes in handy for mincing fresh herbs. Clean the grinder by adding torn white bread to it and processing; the bread will pick up the spice residue.

Fat separator. A fat separator looks something like a measuring cup, but it has a spout that starts at the bottom. It's great for defatting home-made stock. The fat floats to the top of the separator, so you can simply pour off the lean liquid underneath.

Hot-air popcorn popper. Popcorn is an ideal snack—provided it's not made in oil and coated with butter. A hot-air popper doesn't use oil, and the popcorn it produces has less fat, less sodium, and fewer calories than store-bought microwave popcorn.

Kitchen scale. A scale comes in handy when you're trying to figure out portion sizes. You want one that can weigh ounces.

Nonstick pots and pans. Cookware with a non-stick coating allows you to prepare foods with little or no added fat. Be aware that some nonstick coatings scratch easily—and once they're damaged, they lose effectiveness. For this reason, you should use only wooden or plastic utensils when cooking. Some newer nonstick pots and pans have improved coatings that are guaranteed to last for at least 20 years. They also come in all shapes and sizes. The 10-inch and 12-inch skillets are the most versatile, so you may want to start your collection with them and add on as necessary.

Slow cooker. In a slow cooker, lean meats simmer in their own juices for a long period, so they

Smart Cooking

How you prepare food can make all the difference in its healthfulness. Creamed or sautéed fish can cancel out all good intentions; boiled broccoli loses a great deal of its superior nutritional edge. The following cooking methods help preserve food's nutrients while keeping fat and calories to a minimum.

Baking. Meats, fish, and poultry retain their distinctive flavors when baked. To prevent food from drying out, cover it for part of the baking time.

Braising. Simmering food in liquid in a moderately hot oven works exceptionally well for tenderizing lean cuts of meat and dense vegetables such as potatoes and carrots. Fat seeps out of the food into the cooking liquid, where you can skim it off.

Broiling. The food is placed on a broiler rack, which allows the fat to drain into the pan below. Use this method to prepare lean meats, poultry, and fish.

Grilling. Broiling and grilling have similar benefits,

become as tender as their fatty counterparts. This appliance is also ideal for preparing foods with long cooking times, such as soups, stews, and beans.

Steamer. Steaming isn't just for vegetables anymore. This versatile cooking method also produces great-tasting meats, poultry, and fish. It takes less time than boiling, and it does a better job of preserving a food's nutrients and flavor. You can choose a stainless steel or bamboo steamer to use with other cookware, or a freestanding electric model.

nutrition-wise. The main difference: With broiling, the food is under the heat source, but with grilling, the food cooks over the heat.

Microwaving. Sure, it saves time. But microwaving also saves nutrients—not to mention flavor.

Poaching. Food simmers in liquid—such as water, broth, or juice—for a short period of time. It's ideal for preparing fish and boned poultry, as well as fragile fruits such as pears.

Roasting. Like baking, roasting uses dry heat. Help keep the food moist by basting it with broth, fruit juice, or low-fat marinade.

Steaming. The healthy alternative to boiling, steaming preserves nutrients because the food is cooked over water rather than in it.

Stir-frying. Any combination of vegetables becomes a meal in minutes with this quick cooking method. Try using water, defatted broth, or citrus juice instead of oil for an even healthier stir-fry.

Stove-top grill. Enjoy grilling year-round by bringing it indoors. This type of grill fits right over one or two burners on your stove. Use it to make meats, fish, and vegetables without extra fat or oil.

Wok. If you enjoy stir-fries, a wok is your cookware of choice. It cooks quickly, so foods retain their nutrients, but it requires only a small amount of oil. Choose one with a nonstick surface and a lid. And for the best heat conduction on American gas and electric ranges, buy a wok with a flat bottom.

Recipe Makeovers

Make Old Favorites Healthy

A very famous French TV chef who shall remain anonymous once told a group of food writers that "low-fat food is an oxymoron."

"What's the point in eating food if you take all the fat out of it?" she trilled. "Fat *is* where you find the flavor."

Sorry, Chef, but we're about to prove you wrong. Low-fat food has suffered long enough from its reputation of being bland, boring, and tasteless. Great chefs all over the country are betting their reputations on creations brimming with flavor and devoid of fat.

So how do you make great-tasting food—the favorite foods you and your family love to eat—without all the fat? It really isn't all that hard. All you need to know is how to substitute a little of this for a little of that.

Look on the Light Side

Revamping a recipe to cut down on fat is not an exact science. You'll have to do some tinkering to find the "formula" that meets your standards for both fat content and taste. Your best bet is to make just one change to a recipe at a time, advises Evelyn Tribole, R.D., author of *Healthy Homestyle Cooking* and *Eating on the Run*. That way, if the dish doesn't turn out quite as you expected, it's much easier to troubleshoot. Be sure to take notes on your change and the result. If it turns out well, you can incorporate another fat-reducing change the next time you make it.

Here are some fat-paring pointers from the pros to help you cook up your own lean cuisine.

Know your fat facts. Oils are pure fat, so you should skimp on them as much as possible when you cook. But just as important as how much you use is which kind you use. Butter is high in saturated fat, which you should avoid. Instead use canola, olive, and peanut oils. These are high in monounsaturated fat, which is better for you.

Incidentally, don't pour oil straight into the pan. Instead, put some into a spray bottle, then give the pan a squirt. "People do use less oil with a spray," notes Franca Alphin, R.D., nutrition director at the Duke University Diet and Fitness Center in Durham, North Carolina. "Remember, 1 second of spraying equals 7 calories."

Skip the oil in sautés. Instead of sautéing vegetables in oil, switch to water, fruit juice, or nonfat vegetable, chicken, or beef broth. Besides cutting down on added fat, these cooking liquids do a better job than oil of playing up a food's natural flavors.

Rethink meat choices. "In most cases, you can substitute turkey for red meat in recipes without making any other changes," says Joanne D'Agostino, a low-fat cooking consultant in Easton, Pennsylvania. For example, ground skinless turkey breast works well in meat loaf, chili, and spaghetti sauce.

If you have a casserole recipe that calls for ground beef, replace half the beef with cooked brown rice, bulgur, couscous, or chopped beans. You'll reduce the fat content of the dish—and you'll get a healthy dose of fiber.

Whip up a dream cream. Recipes for soups

Smart Substitutes

A little culinary sleight of hand goes a long way in cutting the fat content of your favorite recipes—and saving them from mealtime extinction. By exchanging high-fat ingredients for leaner alternatives, like those listed below, you can keep on eating the foods you love. And just look at the grams of fat you'll save!

Instead of . . .	Use . . .	And Cut the Fat by . . .
½ cup oil (for baking)	½ cup applesauce	109 g
½ cup oil (for salad dressing)	½ cup unsweetened pineapple juice	109 g
½ cup margarine or butter (for baking)	½ cup baby food prunes	92 g
½ cup margarine or butter (for frosting)	½ cup marshmallow cream	92 g
8 oz cream cheese	8 oz nonfat ricotta cheese	79 g

and sauces often use cream, egg yolks, and other high-fat ingredients as thickeners. Substitute healthier pureed cooked vegetables, such as carrots, potatoes, or cauliflower.

In a bisque soup, use buttermilk, nonfat half-and-half, or evaporated skim milk instead of heavy cream.

Instead of . . .	Use . . .	And Cut the Fat by . . .
1 cup cream	1 cup evaporated skim milk	60 g
1 cup sour cream	1 cup nonfat yogurt	40 g
4 oz full-fat Cheddar cheese	4 oz nonfat Cheddar cheese	38 g
1 cup whole-milk ricotta cheese	1 cup 1-percent-fat cottage cheese	30 g
3 oz 80-percent-lean ground beef	3 oz ground skinless turkey breast	17 g
1 Tbsp full-fat mayonnaise	1 Tbsp nonfat mayonnaise	11 g
1 cup whole milk	1 cup skim milk	8 g
3 oz canned oil-packed light tuna	3 oz canned water-packed light tuna	6 g
1 whole egg	2 egg whites	5 g
1 oz unsweetened baking chocolate	3 Tbsp cocoa powder plus 2 tsp vegetable oil	4 g

(Although its name makes it sound fatty, buttermilk is actually equal to 1 percent low-fat milk in terms of fat content.)

Bake better goodies. Slim down cakes, muffins, and other sweet treats by replacing the shortening with fruit-based butter and oil replacement, which you'll find with the cooking oils in the supermarket. Applesauce, mashed bananas, or canned pumpkin can also be used to replace some of the fat. Start by cutting the amount of shortening in half and making up the difference with the fruit substitute. Continue reducing the amount of shortening and increasing the amount of fruit substitute until you find a proportion that produces a taste and texture you like.

Favorites with a Big Fat Difference

Now that you know the basics, you can transform virtually any food into a lean and luscious version of its former fat-laden self. To give you a head start, the country's top nutritionists and chefs have provided their healthy remakes of some popular dishes. Try your hand at these favorites—and discover just how easy revamping recipes can be.

Beef stroganoff. Canned cream of mushroom soup is a traditional ingredient in stroganoff. Replace it with a reduced-fat version of the soup. Or try this suggestion from Evelyn Tribole: Mix an envelope of onion-mushroom soup mix with 1 cup of evaporated skim milk and 1 tablespoon of cornstarch. Bring to a boil, add cooked, browned beef, then ladle the mixture over noodles.

Brownies. Slim down these treats by using unsweetened cocoa instead of semisweet chocolate, and pureed prunes instead of butter, recommends Susan Purdy, author of *Have Your Cake and Eat It, Too*. "The prunes keep the brownies moist, and the overall fat content is about one-fifth of the fat in a traditional brownie recipe," Purdy says. And by using nonstick spray to "grease" the pan, you'll save even more grams of fat.

Burgers. Even extra-lean ground round—the "healthiest" choice—isn't so healthy after all: Just 3 ounces, broiled and well-drained, has almost 14 grams of fat. But you don't have to give up your beloved burgers—replace some of the ground beef with shredded vegetables (such as carrots, onions, and green peppers) or with mashed pinto or black beans.

Cheesecake. Cottage cheese gives cheesecake a wonderfully smooth texture but without all the fat of cream cheese. Drain it to remove excess liquid, then puree it in a food processor until it's the consistency of sour cream, Purdy says. She also suggests reducing the number of eggs you use. If your recipe calls for three whole eggs, for example, switch to one whole egg plus two egg whites.

Chocolate cake. Slice the fat from this favorite by using less butter or shortening—say, ⅔ cup instead of 1 cup, Purdy suggests. Then go one step further by replacing a small portion of the remaining butter or shortening with nonfat or low-fat plain yogurt.

Clam chowder. If you're accustomed to adding bacon to your chowder, try a couple of drops of liquid smoke instead, Tribole says. She also suggests using low-fat (1 percent) milk instead of whole milk and evaporated skim milk instead of cream.

Fettuccine sauce. Traditional recipes for this favorite pasta topping call for butter, heavy cream, and Parmesan cheese. For a trim and tasty imitation, blend nonfat cream cheese, skim milk, and nonfat cottage cheese in a food processor for about 4 minutes, then warm the mixture, says Lynn Fischer, author of *Fabulous Fat-Free Cooking*. If you like, add ¼ cup of very lean diced ham and 1 cup of peas.

French fries. Cut unpeeled potatoes—or sweet potatoes, for a new twist on an old favorite—into ½-inch-thick slices. Coat the slices with a mixture of low-sodium soy sauce and a few drops of dark sesame oil. Then grill or broil the "fries" until they turn crisp and golden.

French toast. Skip the whole eggs and dip your bread in egg substitute instead, Fischer suggests. And don't slather your French toast with butter—stick with a small amount of maple syrup.

Fried chicken. Remake a high-fat standby with this suggestion from Marilyn Cerino, R.D., nutrition consultant at the Benjamin Franklin Center for Health of Pennsylvania Hospital in Philadelphia. Dip boneless, skinless chicken breasts in a mixture of skim milk and egg whites, then roll them in either bread crumbs or seasoned flour. Coat a nonstick pan with nonstick spray, add 1 teaspoon of olive or canola oil, and flash-fry the chicken over medium-high heat for 30 seconds on each side to make it crispy. Then bake at 400°F for five minutes, or until the chicken is cooked through.

Lasagna. Lighten up this Italian classic by substituting a mixture of extra-lean ground beef and ground turkey breast for the usual high-fat sausage. Even better: Layer the noodles with roasted or grilled vegetables, such as eggplant or zucchini, says Julia Della Croce, author of *The Vegetarian Table*. And use nonfat ricotta cheese rather than the full-fat variety.

Manicotti. For manicotti filling, process nonfat cottage cheese in a food processor for a few seconds. It works just as well as full-fat ricotta cheese, according to D'Agostino. You can make the filling even healthier by mixing the cottage cheese with frozen spinach that has been thawed and squeezed dry.

Meat loaf. Make your meat loaf with extra-lean ground beef and replace half the usual amount with a packaged soy meat substitute, Fischer says. Then add chopped onions, celery, carrots, mushrooms, green peppers, or the whites of hard-boiled eggs to keep the loaf moist. And if your recipe calls for whole eggs, use just egg whites instead.

Muffins. Most muffin recipes call for oil. You can get away with half the amount by replacing half the oil with drained applesauce or pureed prunes, says Jeanne Jones, "Cook It Light" syndicated columnist and author of *Healthy Cooking for People Who Don't Have Time to Cook*. To eliminate the fat altogether, try fruit-based butter and oil replacement.

Pie. Phyllo dough makes a perfect pie crust, with a lot less fat than a regular crust, Cerino says. Cut three sheets of phyllo in half. Lay one piece across a 9-inch pie plate and press it into place. Fold any overhanging dough toward the center of the plate, crumpling it slightly to make it fit. Mist the phyllo with nonstick spray. Repeat this process with the remaining pieces. Then bake the crust at 375°F for 4 to 6 minutes, or until golden. Add fresh fruit, such as strawberries, just before serving, Cerino suggests.

Pizza. These days, many "gourmet" pizzas skip the cheese entirely, D'Agostino notes. You don't have to eliminate it from your homemade pies, though— just switch to a low-fat variety and use only about 2 ounces. And replace high-fat toppings such as sausage and pepperoni with grilled vegetables such as zucchini, peppers, and eggplant.

Potato salad. Slim down this summertime standby by switching to nonfat or low-fat mayonnaise and using just the whites of hard-boiled eggs rather than the whole eggs, Fischer says. You can also boost the salad's taste and texture by adding chopped Spanish onions, celery, dill pickles, and scallions.

Quiche. Quiche recipes traditionally call for a high-fat combination of milk, eggs, and cheese. You can reduce the fat content of this dish considerably by using skim milk, egg substitute (¼ cup for each whole egg), and shredded low-fat cheese.

Sloppy joes. Extra-lean ground beef or ground turkey breast works just as well as regular ground round. Spice up the flavor by combining ½ cup of chunky salsa with a can of tomato sauce.

Spaghetti. Skip the meat sauce and create your own flavorful low-fat spaghetti topping by combining chopped fresh tomatoes, basil, garlic, and a touch of balsamic vinegar. For a meaty texture, use crumbled-up soy burgers or veggie burgers instead of the usual ground beef.

Stuffing. Holiday feasts just wouldn't be the same without stuffing. Make it low-fat with this recipe from Tribole: Sauté chopped onions, celery, and mushrooms in a nonstick skillet that you've coated with nonstick spray. Combine the vegetables with unseasoned cornbread stuffing in a 2-quart casserole, then add some defatted chicken broth to moisten the mixture. Bake at 350°F for 30 to 40 minutes.

Tuna noodle casserole. The tuna and noodles aren't so bad—it's the rest of the casserole that packs the fat. Make yours lean by substituting evaporated skim milk for whole milk and using reduced-fat versions of the canned cream of mushroom soup and the cheese. Also, be sure to choose tuna that's packed in water rather than oil.

Supermarket Smarts

Top Choices in Every Aisle

A foray into one of today's huge grocery stores can make you long for a time gone by, when you simply asked the man behind the counter for a box of cereal and he handed you one. Instead, you have to choose from among literally hundreds of brands, comparing cost, taste, and nutritional value. And that's just for one item. The average supermarket carries about 30,000 different products, edible and nonedible. And every one of them is screaming, "Buy me!"

Short of moving to your own Green Acres and home-growing all your own food, there's not much you can do to avoid the grocery gauntlet. You have to eat, which means you have to buy food. So how do you make your visits to the mega-supermarket more pleasant and productive—and ensure that you arrive home with precisely those items that will do your body good?

You need a plan—an aisle-by-aisle shopping guide to help you bypass the bad stuff and fill your cart with good-for-you foods. "To eat healthy, you need to buy healthy," notes Bonnie Tandy Leblang, R.D., author of the nationally syndicated column "Supermarket Sampler" and six cookbooks, including *Beans: Seventy-*

Nine Recipes for Beans, Lentils, Peas, Peanuts, and Other Legumes. "Smart supermarket shopping strategies are the key to eating well at home."

Shopping à la Cart

It would be nice to think that the supermarket you frequent shares your concerns about good nutrition. To some extent, it probably does. Many chain stores have instituted consumer education programs, posting signs and distributing pamphlets that detail the nutritional values of specific items.

Still, their bottom line is—well, the bottom line. They want you to spend—and to leave the store with more items than the two or three you originally planned to buy. And so they invest literally billions of dollars in dizzying, dazzling displays designed to make the most of every selling opportunity.

You can outwit such temptations and stay true to your healthy eating habits by learning a few grocery ground rules. Here's what the experts recommend.

Don't be list-less. A shopping list is your most important navigational tool for the supermarket. It keeps you focused, minimizes impulse buys, and ensures that you leave the store with exactly what you went in for.

If you seldom have time to write down what you need, create a master list of the items that you most often buy and photocopy it. Then you can simply check off items as they run low.

Clip carefully. Coupons appeal to your money-saving side, but they may not be a nutrition bargain. Be wary of discounted items that don't support healthy eating habits. If you come across a coupon for a new product that you think you'd like to try, take a good look at its nutrition label before buying. Look for low-fat items, which provide less than 3 grams of fat per serving, or items that provide at least 10 percent of the recommended amount of either vitamin A, vitamin C, iron, or calcium (or meet both criteria).

Fill your tank first. "Never, ever, ever shop on an empty stomach," notes Michele Tuttle, R.D., former director of consumer affairs for the Food Marketing Institute in Washington, D.C. "If you're hungry, you'll always buy things that you didn't intend to, and everything will always look more appealing."

This doesn't mean that you have to plan every shopping trip around breakfast, lunch, or dinner. Just munching on an apple or a banana can tide you over, says Debra Waterhouse, R.D., author of *Outsmarting the Female Fat Cell* and *Why Women Need Chocolate*.

Go it alone. It's best not to turn grocery shopping into a social event with a friend—or, for that matter, to take along kids. Either way, you're more inclined to end up with unhealthy foods that you wouldn't otherwise buy.

Watch the clock. Shopping when you're pressed for time or when the supermarket is crowded sets the stage for hasty, unhealthy food decisions. Plan your supermarket runs for off-peak hours. Go on a weekday rather than a weekend, either early in the morning or late in the evening. (With so many chain stores now open 24 hours, you can shop at 3:00 A.M., if you're so inclined.) Just allow yourself plenty of time, so you can read labels carefully and choose foods wisely.

Don't go for come-ons. Supermarkets strategically position every single product to maximize its "sell-ability." Nothing is left to chance—every item in the store has a reason for being placed in a certain aisle, on a certain shelf, and at a certain height. Among the techniques you should be wary of are end-of-aisle displays (sometimes called end caps), which showcase specially priced items; cross-merchandising displays, which pair complementary products like potato chips and soda; and checkout-lane displays, which encourage last-minute impulse purchases.

Skip the samples. You already know how full-fat Swiss cheese tastes, so just say no when someone asks you to make like a gustatory guinea pig. Passing up a 1½-ounce chunk of cheese means sparing yourself a whopping 160 calories and over 11 grams of fat.

Think small. Don't buy those gargantuan family-size and economy-size packages of food unless you really need that much. For one thing, you may end up throwing a lot of it away because of spoilage—which means that you really don't save any money on the purchase. For another, a series of studies at the University of Pennsylvania in Philadelphia has shown that people tend to use more of a food at a time if it comes in a larger package.

Don't ponder the possibilities. The phrase "just in case"—as in "just in case company drops by" or "just in case the kids want something sweet"—has scuttled many attempts at eating right. Shop with only you and your immediate family in mind, not some phantom guests who may or may not show up on your doorstep. And even if they do, you can serve them the same delicious, nutritious foods that you already have on hand.

Just the Facts, Ma'am

Compared with labels of five years ago, the ones we see these days present a veritable *Encyclopaedia Britannica* of nutrition information. An ingredients list and a Nutrition Facts chart graces nearly every packaged food, as well as many fresh foods. They tell you not only what a particular product is made from but also how much of certain nutrients it contains. That way, you can decide whether that product has a place in your healthy diet.

Of course, you have to know how to interpret all those servings, percentages, and 10-syllable chemical names. Here's a short primer on what they mean and what to look for.

Serving size. According to the Food and Drug Administration, which regulates food labeling, the serving size reflects the portion that people *actually* eat. You have to ask yourself whether this amount of food seems realistic. If you think you consume more or less—if you have, say, four cookies instead of the serving size of two—then the rest of the figures in the Nutrition Facts chart won't hold up. In the case of the cookies, you'd be getting twice as much of everything listed in the chart.

Percent Daily Value. This column of the Nutrition Facts chart shows how a food helps you meet your daily nutrient needs. The percentages are calculated for a 2,000-calorie-a-day diet. If you're eating smaller portions and fewer total calories overall—as many women do—you'll get smaller amounts of the nutrients as well.

To quickly assess a food's nutritional value, use these rules of thumb from the American Dietetic Association. For total fat, cholesterol, and sodium, each Percent Daily Value should not exceed 100 percent—and the lower, the better. For fiber, vitamins A and C, calcium, and iron, higher Percent Daily Values are ideal. (In general, food labels list only these four vitamins and minerals plus fiber because people tend to not get enough of them.)

Calories and total fat. These figures come in handy if you're counting calories and grams of fat. For example, if a food contains one-third of the fat in your

(continued on page 94)

91

The Real Meaning of Lite

Behind every low-this and reduced-that is a standardized definition developed by the Food and Drug Administration and the U.S. Department of Agriculture. Here's a sampling of some commonly used label lingo and the nutritional information that it represents.

Sugar-free	Contains less than 0.5 gram of sugar per serving
Calorie-free	Contains fewer than 5 calories per serving
Low-calorie	Contains 40 or fewer calories per serving
Reduced-calorie	Contains 25 percent fewer calories than the regular product
Fat-free	Contains less than 0.5 gram of fat per serving
Low-fat	Contains 3 grams or less of fat per serving
Reduced-fat	Contains no more than 75 percent of the fat found in regular versions or comparable food
Light or lite	Contains one-third fewer calories or half the fat of the regular food
Cholesterol-free	Contains less than 2 milligrams of cholesterol and 2 grams or less of saturated fat per serving

Low-cholesterol	Contains 20 milligrams or less of cholesterol, 2 grams or less of saturated fat, and 13 grams or less of total fat per serving
Reduced-cholesterol	Contains 75 percent or less of the cholesterol found in the regular food and 2 grams or less of saturated fat per serving
Sodium-free	Contains less than 5 milligrams of sodium per serving
Very low sodium	Contains less than 35 milligrams of sodium per serving
Low-sodium	Contains 140 milligrams or less of sodium per serving
Reduced-sodium	Contains no more than 75 percent of the sodium found in the regular food
Extra-lean	Meat, seafood, or poultry that has less than 2 grams of saturated fat, less than 5 grams of total fat, and less than 95 milligrams of cholesterol per 3-ounce serving
Lean	Meat, seafood, or poultry that has 4.5 grams or less of saturated fat, less than 10 grams of total fat, and less than 95 milligrams of cholesterol per 3-ounce serving

daily budget, keep that in mind for the rest of the day so that you don't go over your budget.

Saturated fat and cholesterol. A diet high in either of these may increase your risk of a serious health problem such as heart disease or cancer. So look for low numbers here. You shouldn't get more than 7 percent of your daily calories from saturated fat. For example, if you're eating 2,000 calories a day, no more than 140 calories should come from saturated fat. Count up the saturated fat listed on nutrient labels for everything you eat, and limit it to 15 grams a day. (A gram of fat has 9 calories.) As for cholesterol, the American Heart Association recommends consuming no more than 300 milligrams a day.

Sodium. Limit your daily intake of sodium to under 2,400 milligrams per day. High-sodium diets have been linked to high blood pressure.

Dietary fiber. According to the National Cancer Institute, you need to consume between 20 and 30 grams of fiber every day for optimum health.

Ingredients. You'll find this list separate from the Nutrition Facts chart. Be sure to check it out. The ingredients appear in descending order by amount, from most to least. Look for foods with short lists rather than long ones. And make sure that any fat or oil is way down on the list.

Hello, Good Buys

You know the inside scoop on supermarket shopping strategies, and you've learned how to decipher label lingo. You're all set for a nutrition-savvy shopping spree.

To get your trip down the aisles off on the right foot, we asked Elizabeth A. Brown, R.D., nutritionist and weight-control specialist at the Lehigh Valley Hospital Center for Health Promotion and Disease Prevention in Allentown, Pennsylvania, to take you on a personal, guided tour of a typical grocery store. Here are her recommendations for what you should buy and what you should bypass.

Produce

You can't go wrong in this aisle—the bright colors tell you that these foods are loaded with vitamins and minerals. Don't be afraid to experiment with the many exotic fruits and vegetables you find here. Variety and balance are very important to good nutrition, as research continues to uncover "hidden" nutrients in an array of produce. Flavonoids are a good example: These little-known chemical compounds, found in abundance in kale, cranberries, onions, and in the white pulp of citrus fruit, may help reduce your risk of heart disease and cancer.

Best choices: Choose dark green vegetables such as broccoli and kale for fiber, and orange, red, and yellow produce such as carrots, cantaloupe, and sweet potatoes for beta-carotene. Kale has a lot of nutritional value, with healthy doses of vitamins A and C. Other notable nutrient-rich selections include asparagus, oranges, papaya, and green peppers.

Deli

Proceed with caution! Most of what you see in the deli showcase serves up lots of fat and calories, and since the nutrition information is seldom posted for these items, it's hard to know exactly what you're getting. If you want to buy lunch meat, fresh is a better choice than processed. Select only the leanest cuts. Avoid cured meats—they contain nitrites, food preservatives that have been linked to health problems ranging from migraines to cancer. And go easy on the prepared salads. They're usually made with full-fat ingredients.

Best choices: Chicken breast and turkey breast come up winners here. Both are low in fat and excellent sources of niacin and vitamin B_6. In fact, 3 ounces of chicken breast supplies 58 percent of the Daily Value (DV) of niacin for women. You get nice amounts of iron, too.

Breads/Baked Goods

Another dietary danger zone. You're especially vulnerable to impulse purchases in this department when you're tired or shopping on an empty stomach. At times like these, your body craves carbs, and high-fat, high-sugar treats seem especially attractive. Bypass the cakes and doughnuts and head for the whole-grain breads and other baked goods. Read the label for fiber and iron content, and choose items that are enriched and fortified.

Best choices: Bagels are a good source of iron and of the B vitamins niacin, riboflavin, and thiamin. Just watch the serving size. With some of the larger bagels, you could end up consuming a lot more calories than you think. Among breads, whole-grain types are versatile and supply 2 to 3 grams of fiber per slice. Be aware, though, that fiber content varies from one brand of whole-grain bread to the next—and some brands may not even have significant amounts of the nutrient. On the other hand, many "light" versions of breads and English muffins can pack 3 to 6 grams per serving. Read the label to be sure.

Dairy

Here you'll find the cream of the calcium crop. Milk, yogurt, and cheese all weigh in with generous amounts of the mineral. Unfortunately, the regular varieties also have generous amounts of fat. Select leaner alternatives when you can, such as nonfat or low-fat (1 percent) milk and nonfat or low-fat yogurt. Likewise, the healthiest choices in cheese are made from nonfat or low-fat milk and are not highly processed.

As for the margarine-versus-butter debate: Margarine seems better than butter, but it may not be as good as you think. It contains trans-fatty acids, which act like heart-unhealthy saturated fat. Choose light margarine over regular. And it's okay to have a pat of butter once in a while—portion control is what counts.

Best choices: Yogurt supplies even more calcium than milk: A 1-cup serving of the nonfat variety has 488 milligrams, or 49 percent of a woman's recommended daily intake. Look for a brand with active cultures, which may help prevent recurrent yeast infections. Be wary of brands sweetened with aspartame (NutraSweet). Not enough studies have been done to know what effects this ingredient may have on the body.

Pasta, Rice, and Beans

The *Prevention* Food Pyramid for Women says you should eat five 1-ounce servings of protein-rich foods every day. Beans make an excellent protein source, especially if you don't eat a lot of meat. So stock up on all varieties.

Pasta counts toward your daily grain quota of six to nine servings. Opt for dried whole-wheat varieties over fresh, since fresh is usually made with eggs and tends to have more cholesterol and fat. Whole-wheat varieties are also a great source of fiber.

Roll your cart right past those premixes and heavily prepared foods, like packaged pasta and rice dishes. Besides feeding you a hefty amount of fat, they offer little nutritional value.

Best choices: Beans, beans, beans. They pack a nutritional punch of protein, fiber, iron, and folate, and they're filling and versatile to boot. And don't forget rice. One-half cup of the brown variety, in particular, supplies some fiber and the B vitamins B_6, niacin, and thiamin in exchange for no cholesterol and just a smidgen of fat. You may also want to try bulgur. It has even more fiber than rice, no cholesterol, and practically no fat.

Cookies and Crackers

Crackers are an okay snack, as long as you pay attention to how many you're eating. Most people eat between 10 and 12 at a time, which exceeds the typical serving size. Cookies of any kind should be reserved for an occasional treat, since they're nutritionally empty.

Best choices: Look for whole-wheat crackers that contain no more than 3 grams of fat per serving. Also check out the animal crackers and graham crackers. All of these are cholesterol-free and low-fat, too.

Snack Foods

Pick up some popcorn for a filling snack that provides a bit of fiber. Just read the label to make sure it's low-fat. If it's something sweet you're after, opt for marshmallows, gummy candies, or jelly beans. None of these has any nutritional value, but they do have a lot less fat than most candies. Check out the ingredient list on the package. The shorter it is, the fewer additives the item contains.

Best choices: Besides popcorn, smart snack selections include pretzels, flavored rice cakes, and sunflower seeds. Honey-mustard pretzels tend to have more fat than regular varieties, so go easy on them. Sunflower seeds also have a lot of fat (most of it unsaturated), so they're not for everyday munching.

Canned Foods

Fruits and vegetables. Canned produce has at least one advantage over fresh: It has a longer shelf life. It also helps ensure that you're meeting the six- to seven-serving quota for fruits and veggies (one vitamin C, one folate, two phytochemicals, one carotenoid, one to two fiber) that's recommended in the *Prevention* Food Pyramid for Women.

Although some vitamins can be lost in the canning process, one University of Illinois analysis found that some canned fruits and vegetables, like pineapple and carrots, contain as much of vitamins A and C as the fresh or frozen varieties. Because they're canned without their skins, however, they don't have quite as much fiber as their fresh and frozen counterparts. Look for products that are packed in water or light syrup, with little or no added sugar.

Best choices: Among canned fruits, choose chunky applesauce, mandarin oranges, peaches, and pears. Healthy selections among canned vegetables include kale, asparagus, green beans, spinach, and yams.

Soups. Depending on what kind you choose, soup serves up an array of nutrient-dense vegetables in every spoonful. It's a simple, satisfying way to boost your consumption of these good-for-you foods. Choose nonfat or low-fat products, taking note of the serving size. Sometimes it's smaller than people think. Skip the cream soups.

Best choices: Black bean soup offers a good amount of iron—about 2 milligrams, or 12 percent of the DV—but very little fat and no cholesterol. Lentil soup, another low-fat selection, is also an impressive source of iron (3 milligrams, or 14 percent of the DV) as well as folate (50 micrograms, or 12.5 percent of the DV).

Meats and Poultry

There are three grades, or qualities, of beef sold in most supermarkets. Prime cuts have the most fat, select cuts have the least, and choice cuts fall somewhere in between. You want to look for cuts stamped select. The less marbling a piece of meat has, the leaner it is.

Choose chicken pieces labeled "extra-lean" or "lean." White meat is a healthier choice than dark, but dark meat has more iron and zinc, so you don't necessarily want to completely eliminate it from your diet. Do be very cautious with ground chicken, though. The high-fat skin may have been mixed in with the meat during processing. Check the label for fat content or ask the butcher to grind some plain chicken breasts for you.

When serving meat or poultry, remember to stick with a 3-ounce portion. That's roughly the size of a deck of cards or about the size of the palm of your hand.

Best choices: Chicken breast and turkey breast have less than half the fat of most cuts of meat. Among meats, pork tenderloin is among the leanest cuts, as are select-grade bottom and top round.

Seafood

Almost any fish or shellfish you can think of has nutritional benefit. Some, like Atlantic herring, canned salmon, fresh tuna, and Atlantic mackerel, are rich in omega-3 fatty acids. Medical evidence indicates that omega-3's can reduce heart-unhealthy triglycerides, inhibit the growth of breast cancer cells, and even prevent gallstones. Some seafood does contain fat, but it's not enough to raise the level of cholesterol in your blood. Shellfish are a good example: They don't have a lot of saturated fat, which is the real culprit in raising blood cholesterol levels. Do steer clear of prepared seafood salads, though. They're bound to be loaded with fat.

Best choices: In addition to being a top-notch source of omega-3's, canned salmon (with bones) delivers roughly 20 percent of your recommended daily calcium intake in a 3-ounce serving. Fresh salmon, while not as rich in omega-3's as the canned kind, contains a wealth of B vitamins. You get over 80 percent of the DV of B_{12}, along with lots of niacin and some riboflavin, thiamin, and B_6. Fresh tuna is also a stellar source of these B vitamins, supplying almost one-third of the DV of B_{12}. White- and light-meat tuna, canned in water, are low-fat, high-protein staples that you shouldn't pass up.

Cereals

No matter what you choose in this aisle, you really can't lose. Even sugary cereals fulfill roughly one-quarter of your nutrient needs for an entire day. That's because cereals are fortified. Still, you should compare sugar contents and pick the product that has less.

You can't beat cereal as a fiber source, either. In fact, some products have as much as 13 grams of fiber per serving, nearly three-quarters of the minimum recommended daily intake.

Best choices: Top fiber sources in the cereal aisle include Fiber One from General Mills (14 grams per ½ cup) and Kellogg's All-Bran (almost 10 grams per ½ cup). Also check out the various brands of raisin bran and anything whole-grain.

Condiments

Oils. All oils are 100 percent fat. What differs is their proportions of monounsaturated, polyunsaturated, and saturated fats. You want an oil that is high in monounsaturates and low in saturates. Spray oils work well because they have built-in portion control. Rather than spending more money for the fancy packaging, you can make your own spray oil by pouring oil into a spray bottle.

Best choices: Canola oil has the best fat profile. Of its 14 grams of fat, 8 are monounsaturated, while only 1 is saturated. Olive oil has a high monounsaturated fat content, too, but it also has a strong flavor, so it's not usually recommended for baking.

Salad dressings. Dressings don't have a lot to offer nutritionally, but at least they get people to eat their veggies. Pay attention to serving size: The label usually says 1 to 2 tablespoons, but most folks use a lot more. You can add flavored vinegar to an oil-based dressing to reduce its fat content. If it's a non-oil-based dressing, just add water.

Best choices: Dressings with an oil-and-vinegar base have less sugar and additives than dressings that are creamy. If you're making your own, try red-wine, raspberry, or balsamic vinegar. Their robust flavors mean you can go easy on the oil—and they have very little sugar and fat. Light mayo has better flavor than the nonfat variety.

Frozen Foods

Believe it or not, frozen produce has a nutritional advantage over fresh. Because the fruits and veggies are in a deep freeze, they retain the nutrients that fresh varieties lose as they age. Since you don't know how long fresh produce has been on display, you can't be sure that you're getting all of its nutrients. Try a variety of frozen fruits and veggies for a healthy mix of vitamins and minerals.

The rest of the frozen foods aisle is a mixed bag, nutrition-wise. There are some decent heat-and-serve foods, like pizzas and microwavable dinners. But you have to watch their calorie and fat content. In general, steer clear of anything that's breaded because it has added fat. And try to limit your intake of frozen foods that contain more than 5 grams of fat per serving.

Ice cream is okay as an occasional treat. A 1-cup serving has nearly 20 percent of the DV for calcium. Just be sure to pay attention to the serving size when you indulge. One cup of vanilla ice cream also has 270 calories and 14 grams of fat, making half of those calories come from fat.

Best choices: Among frozen vegetables, asparagus, broccoli, and spinach all deliver a diverse array of nutrients. Pick up some pierogies: They're low in fat, as long as you prepare them by boiling, microwaving, or pan-frying with spray oil. Soft pretzels make a good low-fat snack, too—but check out the serving size before buying.

The Salad Trap

A Good Thing Gone Bad?

When you're ordering at your favorite restaurant, a trip to the salad bar may seem like a more virtuous choice than a burger. But if you garnish your greens with the wrong toppings, you might as well eat the ground round—with fries on the side.

To its credit, a salad is an easy way to boost your

Sizing Up the Salads

A salad isn't always the healthiest choice on a restaurant menu. Depending on what's in it, it can have an even worse nutritional profile than fast food.

Below is the nutrient content of four popular main-dish salads, based on serving sizes of 2 to 3½ cups—typical of the humongous portions that many restaurants serve.

Chef Salad

Description: A large bed of greens heaped with ham, salami, and chicken breast and garnished with eggs, tomatoes, cucumbers, carrots, Cheddar cheese, and Gruyère cheese. Served with ranch dressing.
Per 3-cup serving:
  Calories: 743
  Fat: 48 grams; 59 percent of calories
  Cholesterol: 389 milligrams
  Sodium: 1,340 milligrams

Grilled Chicken Caesar Salad

Description: Romaine lettuce, anchovies, garlic, Parmesan cheese, croutons, olive oil, and lemon juice, topped with slices of grilled chicken breast.
  Per 3- to 3½-cup serving:
  Calories: 941

daily intake of vegetables and fruits. You should eat at least six servings of produce every day, and 1 cup of raw, leafy vegetables counts as a serving, as does ½ cup of chopped raw vegetables, berries, or cut-up fruit. Based on these amounts, a typical main-dish salad

Fat: 46 grams; 44 percent of calories
Cholesterol: 114 milligrams
Sodium: 2,342 milligrams

Salade Niçoise

Description: Grilled marinated fresh tuna on a bed of mixed greens with green beans, onions, potatoes, tomatoes, eggs, anchovies, capers, and black olives. Served with French vinaigrette. (Don't let the word *vinaigrette* fool you—its base is olive oil.)
Per 2-cup serving:
Calories: 680
Fat: 48 grams; 64 percent of calories
Cholesterol: 236 milligrams
Sodium: 860 milligrams

Taco Salad

Description: Mounds of lettuce topped with simmering ground beef, black beans, pinto beans, tomatoes, onions, Monterey Jack cheese, olives, salsa, and sour cream served in a tortilla shell.
Per 3-cup serving:
Calories: 886
Fat: 62 grams; 63 percent of calories
Cholesterol: 112 milligrams
Sodium: 539 milligrams

could probably get you as much as halfway toward your six-a-day goal.

What's more, all those veggies and fruits often contain loads of nutrients that your body needs, such as vitamins A and C, folate, and fiber. And many are rich in phytochemicals, disease-fighting, health-promoting chemical compounds that scientists have just begun to isolate in foods.

Unfortunately, the natural goodness of these ingredients is routinely undermined by the fat we pour on top to make it all taste good. "Salad dressing is the biggest source of fat in a person's diet," notes Jayne Hurley, R.D., senior nutritionist with the Center for Science in the Public Interest, a nonprofit consumer group in Washington, D.C., and a writer for *Nutrition Action Healthletter*. In fact, according to statistics from the National Cancer Institute and the U.S. Department of Agriculture Human Nutrition Information Service, salad dressing accounts for almost 10 percent of the average person's fat intake—more than even margarine, cheese, or ground beef.

Then there are the other high-fat salad toppings: olives, croutons, cheeses, bacon bits, and chow mein noodles, to name just a few. Pair them with a ladle or two of creamy dressing, and that formerly nutritious salad can easily surpass the 1,000-calorie mark. By comparison, even a Burger King Double Whopper with Cheese has only 960 calories.

Good Grazing

The salad, of course, has a place in a healthy diet—if you know how to navigate the salad bar. The following tips from nutrition experts can help you create salads that draw the line at fat and calories.

Turn over a new leaf. Iceberg lettuce is standard at most salad bars, but truth be told, it doesn't hold a candle to its darker green brethren in terms of nutrient content. Romaine lettuce, for example, has twice as much calcium and iron and eight times as much vitamin A and vitamin C as iceberg. As a good rule of thumb, the darker your leafy greens, the more nutritious they are. Other smart selections to look for include kale, spinach, watercress, and arugula.

Veg out. Fresh, raw vegetables add flavor and color to a salad, not to mention healthy doses of important vitamins and minerals. You can beef up your salad's nutritional profile with any combination of the following toppings.

♦ Beets: One-half cup of these red gems supplies a whopping 68 micrograms of folate, a vitamin that moms-to-be need to protect their babies against birth defects. There's also evidence to suggest that folate may protect against cervical dysplasia, the development of abnormal cells in the cervix that is sometimes a precursor to cancer.

♦ Broccoli florets: One-half cup provides 41 milligrams of disease-fighting vitamin C, or 68 percent of your Daily Value (DV).

♦ Carrots: You won't find a better food source of vitamin A—½ cup has 17,158 IU, or over 300 percent of the DV. You get a good amount of fiber, too.

♦ Cauliflower: Like its cruciferous cousin broccoli, cauliflower is rich in vitamin C—about 23 milligrams in ½ cup.

♦ Celery: Except for small amounts of folate, vitamin C, fiber, and potassium, celery doesn't have a whole lot of nutritional value. But it does give your salad a lot of crunch and practically no fat for just a few calories.

♦ Cucumbers: Another "crunchable," cucumbers contribute small amounts of fiber, folate, potassium, and vitamin C to your salad.

♦ Mushrooms: Along with copper, mushrooms provide a B-vitamin boost of folate, niacin, and riboflavin.

♦ Peppers: Sweet red peppers are another stellar source of vitamin C, providing 87 milligrams per ½ cup chopped. Their green counterparts supply a not-too-shabby 66 milligrams. You can't beat either variety for vibrant color and satisfying crunch.

♦ Red cabbage: With more vitamin C than the pale green variety, red cabbage also supplies some vitamin B_6 and fiber.

♦ Tomatoes: There's no better source of lycopene, a relatively unknown "supernutrient" that scientists believe helps to protect against a number of different cancers as well as cervical dysplasia.

Be fruit-full. Many salad bars feature nutrient-rich fresh fruits, from melon wedges and pineapple spears to kiwifruit and berries. Enjoy them on the side—or add them to your greens to give your salad just a touch of natural sweetness.

Pick some protein. Scout the salad bar for legumes such as kidney beans, chickpeas, black beans, lentils, and split peas. They're low in fat and high in fiber and protein—perfect as a meat substitute in a salad.

If you have a hankering for the real thing, choose turkey breast or chicken breast. They're not as low in fat as legumes (they get about 20 percent of their calories from fat), but they're not nearly as bad as most lunch meats.

Sprinkle on the cheese. When sprinkled on your salad sparingly, cheese supplies a dose of bone-building calcium. It's best to choose low-fat or nonfat varieties, but you can't always tell what you're getting at a salad bar. Grated Parmesan is usually a safe bet. It's higher than most other cheeses in calcium, and 1 to 2 tablespoons can go a little farther than a shredded type.

Fake out fat. Anything can look healthy when it's surrounded by a sea of greens and veggies. But beware the usual salad bar fat traps: nuts and seeds, sliced olives, croutons, chow mein noodles, and bacon bits. Any of these can sabotage your salad by driving up its calorie and fat content.

Sample with restraint. Just because something is called a salad doesn't mean it's good for you. Take potato salad: Just ½ cup can add 179 calories and 10 grams of fat to your plate. In general, it's a good idea to avoid this and other mayonnaise-based, deli-style concoctions.

But if you do want to sample, wait until your second trip to the salad bar. Fill up on the healthy stuff first, so "just a taste" doesn't turn into an entire plateful.

Dressing Down

Your salad may not seem complete without your favorite dressing drizzled over the top. But before you grab the ladle and pour, consider this: If you overdo it, you can turn a perfectly healthful plate of greens and vegetables into unhealthy fare that gets as much as 70 percent of its calories from fat.

The obvious solution is to stick with a nonfat or low-fat salad dressing, but even that should be used with a light touch. You may want to try one of these options instead.

Give it a squeeze. Lemon or lime juice makes a nice substitute for traditional salad dressing, and it gives your salad a burst of vitamin C to boot. Simply

Better Left Undressed

Those ladles in the salad dressings at the salad bar can hold anywhere from ¾ to 2 ounces. That may not sound like much—until you consider how much fat and calories those ounces contain.

Here's how some popular full-fat dressings measure up in terms of fat content per 2-ounce serving (4 tablespoons).

Dressing	Fat (g)	Calories
Blue cheese	32	308
French	26	268
Italian	28	275
Russian	31	302
Thousand Island	22	234

squeeze a slice or two of the fruit right onto your salad for a light yet zesty taste.

Try something new. If you're an oil-and-vinegar fan, sample some of the more exotic vinegars that some salad bars offer these days, such as balsamic, champagne, raspberry, and white- or red-wine. Their robust flavors mean you can get by with a lot less oil—say, three parts vinegar to only one part oil.

Make your own. At home, you can combine a couple of salad bar staples to create a "dressing" with less fat and fewer calories than their premade counterparts. For example, spoon out some low-fat yogurt and add just enough reduced-calorie mayonnaise to thicken it, then add it to your salad. Or mix just a small amount of low-fat dressing with some low-fat cottage cheese and use that as your salad topping.

Think thin. Among regular, full-fat dressings, thin ones such as French and Italian tend to be better choices than thicker ones such as blue cheese and Thousand Island. This is true not because they have less fat but because they spread more easily, so you can use less.

Keep it on the side. Rather than ladling the dressing right over your salad, put it in a small container. Then lightly dip your fork into the container before spearing your salad. This method gives you better portion control.

Water—
Liquid Gold

Drink to Your Health's Content

In the 1970s, we were singing in *"per-fect har-mo-ny"* to a catchy jingle that wanted us to drink Coke. Years later, we became enchanted by a comely couple being romantic over their cups of

Taster's Choice coffee. Then milk became the commercial drink of choice, with its celebrity-mustached ad campaign.

It's time for water to get its due. After all, water is the only fluid that you truly can't live without. Every cell in your body depends on it to function properly. In fact, your body processes about 2 to 3 quarts a day to transport nutrients to where they're needed, get rid of body wastes, regulate temperature, support chemical reactions, and perform other critical tasks.

That's why drinking water is so important. If you don't replenish your internal water supply, you can easily become dehydrated—which in turn prevents your body from performing as it should. This is more of a problem for women than for men, notes Felicia Busch, R.D., a nutritionist in St. Paul, Minnesota, and a fellow of the American Dietetic Association. Unlike men, women tend to have more body fat than muscle. And body fat doesn't hold water as well as muscle.

Benefits by the Glassful

Clearly, water plays a vital role in keeping all of your body's systems running smoothly. But this versatile nutrient can do a whole lot more for your good health. Here are some examples.

Burn fat. Like other chemical reactions in your body, fat-burning occurs only in the presence of water. And some scientists believe that running low on H_2O can actually cause your body to store fat.

Satisfy your appetite. Water takes up room in your stomach, so you feel full and don't want to eat as much. And you won't find a better "diet drink" than water, with no calories or fat.

Quash cravings. Sometimes what you interpret as a hunger pang is really your body telling you it's thirsty. Try sipping a glass of water before you raid the refrigerator—your urge to eat may subside within minutes.

Combat the effects of stress. Stress can really do a number on your body. Staying hydrated keeps your body's systems in balance and counteracts stress "symptoms" such as perspiration, dry mouth, and heart palpitations.

Fend off fatigue. If you feel like you're running on empty, maybe you need to fill up on fluids. Tiredness is a common—though often unrecognized—sign of dehydration.

Boost your brainpower. Dehydration can also leave you with a bad case of mental fuzzies. In fact, some researchers have suggested that too little water in your body can cause your brain to shrink ever so slightly, affecting your ability to think and concentrate.

Turn back the clock. Instead of spending a small fortune on facial creams and lotions, generously sip Nature's beauty fluid. Water helps fend off wrinkles and other signs of aging, for smooth and supple skin.

Keep your body moving. Your body uses water as a natural lubricant. It cushions your joints and helps them stay limber so you don't stiffen up like a statue.

Douse urinary tract infections. In a survey of 16,000 women, 82 percent named water as the most effective home remedy for bladder infections, the most common type of urinary tract infection (UTI). Doctors agree that drinking plenty of fluids can help flush UTI-causing bacteria out of your system.

Stave off colon cancer. Researchers at the Fred Hutchinson Cancer Research Center in Seattle have uncovered a possible link between water consumption and colon cancer. In a survey they conducted, women who drank more than five glasses of water a day had about half the risk of colon cancer of women who drank less than two glasses of water a day.

Getting Your Fill

To replenish the water your body uses up, you need to drink at least eight 8-ounce glasses of water a day—not Diet Coke, coffee, or other popular drinks. Many bottled beverages on the market contain sodium and caffeine, which are diuretics. You may not notice it, but they'll dehydrate, rather than hydrate, you.

"You do get water through certain foods, too, such as fruits and vegetables, which are about 90 percent water," says Judy E. Marshel, R.D., director of Health Resources in Great Neck, New York. "And your body chips in another ½ cup or so as a by-product of metabolism, your body's calorie-burning mechanism." But you should try to drink 64 ounces of water every day, recommends Marshel.

If downing 64 ounces of water daily seems hard to swallow, relax. Try the following strategies recommended by nutrition experts.

Drink up when you wake up. Start your day with a glass of water to help make up for the fluids you lost while you were sleeping.

Contain yourself. Invest in a 32-ounce container that you can carry with you as you go about your daily business and can refill throughout the day.

Sip, don't gulp. Take just a little bit of water at a time. If you try to down all 64 ounces in one, two, or even three sittings, you'll get tired of it mighty quickly.

Beat thirst to the punch. Don't wait until you feel parched to start sipping. By the time your thirst mechanism kicks in, you're already well on your way to empty. In fact, you can lose as much as 2 percent of your body weight through perspiration or urination before you get the urge to drink something.

Consider the conditions. There are times when you may need to increase your water intake beyond the usual 64 ounces a day. For instance, to stay hydrated during a workout, you should drink a large glass of water 30 to 60 minutes beforehand, then take a few sips every 15 minutes or so while you exercise. Likewise, you should up your ounces of H_2O if you're sick, if you spend a lot of time in a heated or air-conditioned environment, or if you're traveling by plane. (The recirculated air in the cabin of the plane can easily leave you dehydrated.)

To Your Health

Take It Easy with Alcohol

Alcohol has sure come a long way, from social scourge in the Roaring Twenties to acclaimed elixir at the turn of the twenty-first century. Indeed, the news that alcohol can protect against heart disease may have you poised to drink a toast to your favorite spirits.

Not so fast, experts say. While alcoholic beverages may offer some health benefits, they also have some very real risks. "The fact remains that alcohol is a general toxin—in other words, it can travel anywhere in your body because there's nothing to stop it," says Anne Geller, M.D., chief of the Smithers Addiction Treatment and Training Center at St. Luke's–Roosevelt Hospital Center in New York City. "And anywhere it goes, it can potentially cause problems."

This is especially true for women, Dr. Geller explains, because women experience the negative effects of alcohol at much lower levels than men do. By one estimate, the harmful amount of alcohol for women is about 60 percent of the harmful amount of alcohol for men.

Now we're not suggesting that you take to the streets, a one-woman army marching for the return of Prohibition. We are saying that you need to consume booze wisely by weighing the pros and cons before you take your next sip.

The French Connection

Those revolutionary French. They're the ones who flambéed conventional nutrition wisdom a few years back, when researchers determined that folks who live in the land of rich cream sauces and decadent pastries are 2½ times less likely than we Americans to die from heart disease. This, despite the fact that they eat four times as much butter as we do.

The secret to their seemingly Teflon-coated cardiovascular systems? Researchers suspect it has something to do with the red wine that the French savor so much.

Red wine is loaded with natural compounds called flavonoids. Research suggests that these supernutrients may protect the heart in two ways. First, evidence indicates that flavonoids may prevent harmful low-density lipoprotein cholesterol from sticking to artery walls and clogging up the works. And second, flavonoids may stop blood platelets from clumping together and forming dangerous clots.

While red wine has the strongest protective effects, other alcoholic beverages can give your heart a boost, too. Though more research is needed, some studies have shown that any alcohol—whether it's white wine, beer, or a mixed drink—can raise your blood level of high-density lipoprotein cholesterol, the good kind that helps keep your arteries clean.

To Drink or Not to Drink

Once you get past all the heart-health headlines, however, alcohol begins to show a decidedly mean streak. Among the most provocative findings so far: A four-state study of 15,000 women revealed that moderate alcohol consumption—just one drink a day—increases breast cancer risk by 30 to 40 percent.

If you're trying to lose weight, alcohol won't do you any favors, either. For one thing, it contributes a lot of extra calories to your diet—105 in 5 ounces of wine and 150 in a 12-ounce beer. At a rate of just one drink a day, that's more than 700 unwanted calories per week. In just 5 weeks, you'd consume enough calories to gain 1 pound.

What's more, alcohol appears to inhibit your body's fat-burning mechanism and promote fat storage. And it pumps up your appetite: One study at the Mayo Clinic in Rochester, Minnesota, found that people consume about 350 extra calories when they have an alcoholic beverage with their meal.

Excessive alcohol consumption, defined as three or more drinks a day, presents its own set of health problems. For starters, heavy drinking wreaks havoc on women's hormones, according to Dr. Geller. A woman may experience irregular menstrual cycles and, eventually, premature menopause. "Your body composition changes, too," Dr. Geller says. "You gain fat and lose muscle." You become more vulnerable to osteoporosis as alcohol leaches calcium from your bones. Your odds of developing colorectal cancer also jump—perhaps by as much as 78 percent, according to Harvard University researchers.

Smart Sipping

Understandably, all these issues have left many experts reluctant to endorse alcohol consumption as a healthy habit. "The question is not 'Is alcohol safe?' but 'What amount of alcohol is safe?'" Dr. Geller says.

Of course, finding the answer will require a lot more research. In the meantime, if you don't drink, don't start. And if you do drink, keep these guidelines in mind.

Know your limit. Guidelines established by the National Institute of Alcohol and Alcohol Abuse suggest that the average person can safely consume one drink a day without experiencing any ill effects. (A drink, incidentally, is defined as 12 ounces of regular beer, 5 ounces of wine, or a cocktail made with 1½ ounces of 80-proof distilled spirits.)

Some experts advocate a more conservative limit— say, two or three drinks per week, tops. "A woman has to weigh her own benefits and risks," Dr. Geller says. "If you have a family history of breast cancer, then you'd be wise to restrict your alcohol consumption. On the other hand, if breast cancer doesn't run in your family but heart disease does, a drink a day won't hurt."

Wash it down. If you do have a drink, follow it with a glass or two of water, suggests Felicia Busch, R.D., a nutritionist in St. Paul, Minnesota, and a fellow of the American Dietetic Association. The reason: Alcohol is a diuretic, which means that it makes you urinate more frequently. Following up with an H_2O chaser helps replenish lost fluids and prevent dehydration.

Consider the source. Red wine doesn't hold a monopoly on heart-healthy flavonoids. They're plentiful in a variety of foods, including onions, apples, broccoli, tea—and, of course, grapes. So instead of imbibing to get your fill of flavonoids, choose one of these nonalcoholic alternatives instead.

Snack Smarts

Yes, You Can Just Keep On Eating

According to the head-counters who track such things, at least three-quarters of us eat one or more snacks every day. The rest may be missing out on the healthiest dietary habit this side of breakfast.

It seems that the experts have begun to rethink the long-accepted notion that snacking expands your waistline, spoils your appetite, rots your teeth, and commits various other nutritional offenses against your health. Many now believe that between-meal nibbling, combined with smaller versions of the traditional three squares, can keep your body functioning on a more even keel and reduce your risk of some big health problems.

"Your body needs food—its fuel—in moderate doses throughout the day so it always has nutrients available," says Pat Harper, R.D., a nutrition consultant in Pittsburgh. "I find that having four or five 'mini-meals' daily helps most people prevent cravings and ultimately achieve and maintain a healthy weight."

This new way of eating—or "grazing"—has put snacking in the nutritional mainstream. But you have to know how to do it right. "Try thinking of snacks as foods eaten between meals rather than as treats or rewards," suggests Barbara Whedon, R.D., dietitian and nutrition counselor at Thomas Jefferson University Hospital in Philadelphia. "You should choose them just as you would plan a meal—with variety, balance, and moderation in mind."

Big Benefits from Grazing

Researchers have only recently begun investigating the possible health benefits of the small-meals-plus-snacks style of eating. But what they've uncovered so far is quite compelling. Here is just a sampling of what grazing can do for you.

Snacking sends pounds packing. People who want to lose weight often skip breakfast as a way to lower their calorie intakes. Studies have shown that this practice does more harm than good. Not eating your morning meal actually makes you more likely to compensate for the missing calories—and then some—by overeating later in the day. On the other hand, eating small meals and snacks more frequently helps you to manage your appetite better, so you never get too hungry.

Grazing can also keep your metabolism, or calorie-burning mechanism, running high. Your body uses calories when you eat and digest food. By consuming smaller amounts of food more frequently, you can end up burning calories very efficiently. You'll be less likely to gain weight, even though it may seem like you're eating more than you did before.

Snacking fights fatigue. When more than 4 hours go by between meals, your body's energy supply—your blood sugar, or glucose—dips low enough to allow fatigue to set in. Well-timed snacks give your body a steady supply of fuel, so you're at your best physically and mentally throughout the day. Studies have shown that a snack between 2:00 P.M. and 4:00 P.M. can improve cognitive skills such as memory, arithmetic reasoning, reading speed, and attention span, notes Harper.

Snacking combats high cholesterol. Research comparing people who eat six or more mini-meals a day with people who eat the customary three squares has consistently shown lower cholesterol levels in the nibblers. In one study, consuming six mini-meals a day shaved cholesterol levels by 8 percent, which translates to a 16 percent reduction in heart attack risk.

Snacking fends off heart attacks. Whenever you eat, your heart has to pump extra blood to your stomach and intestines to aid the digestive process. Snacking can help reduce your risk of heart attack by keeping your heart's workload during digestion to a minimum.

One study demonstrated that meal size can make a difference in terms of cardiovascular demand. When people ate a 240-calorie meal of corn flakes and skim milk, their hearts pumped an extra 84 quarts of blood over the next 2 hours. When they ate a 720-calorie meal with added sugar, bread, and honey, their hearts pumped an extra 258 quarts of blood—enough to fill your car's gas tank five times over. This might help explain why doctors see an increase in the number of heart attack patients within 24 hours after big holiday meals.

Chews Wisely

Now before you get caught up in the grazing craze, just remember that "snack" does not mean a doughnut at midmorning, potato chips at midafternoon, and rocky road ice cream for a nightcap. Whatever you choose to nosh on, it should be reasonably good for you.

To get in the swing of smart snacking, give these tips a try.

Set up a schedule. Plan to eat a little something every 3 to 4 hours over the course of a day, advises Elizabeth Somer, R.D., author of *Nutrition for Women* and *Food and Mood*. Perhaps the simplest way to do this is to divide each of your usual big meals into two smaller ones. Here's what a typical day's eating might look like.

♦ Breakfast: cereal, milk, and orange juice

♦ Morning snack: bagel or banana

♦ Lunch: turkey sandwich with romaine lettuce, tomato, and nonfat mayo or mustard

♦ Afternoon snack: pretzels or baked sweet potato

♦ Dinner: vegetable-bean soup and two small pumper-
nickel rolls

♦ Evening snack: baked apple crisp with low-fat yogurt

Be careful not to just add snacks on top of your
usual diet. That's a surefire way to gain weight.

Play to your tastebuds. "When we choose a
snack, we often simply grab whatever is closest at
hand," Whedon observes. "We don't think about what
we're really hungry for. And that can lead to overeating
because we're not satisfying our cravings."

In general, she says, a snack feeds a need for
something chewy, crunchy, smooth, creamy, cold,
sweet, salty, or some combination of these qualities. "If
you want creamy and sweet, yogurt may be your perfect choice," she notes. "If you desire crunchy and
cold, try slices of green pepper."

Feed your hunger, not your head. Stress,
boredom, and frustration can all nudge you to nibble
when you're not actually hungry. If you suspect that
your urge to eat is emotion-driven, distract yourself by
taking a walk or listening to music.

Think. It's much too easy to overdo portion size,
cautions Margo Denke, M.D., associate professor of internal medicine at the Center for Human Nutrition at
the University of Texas Southwestern Medical Center
at Dallas. You need to pay attention to every bite, especially if you munch while watching television. Otherwise, you could end up taking in more calories than
when you were eating three meals a day.

Stash a stash. Ensure nutritious snacking wherever you go by keeping a stash in your office, car,
purse, and briefcase. Some foods that make wonderful
travel companions are snack-size boxes of raisins and

The 10 Healthiest Snacks

Looking for something to munch? We've ferreted out 10 noteworthy low-fat noshes recommended by the American Dietetic Association that will more than satisfy your tastebuds while sneaking in generous amounts of some very important nutrients.

Bagel. One 2-ounce enriched bagel supplies 2 milligrams of iron—11 percent of the Daily Value (DV)—along with good doses of the B vitamins niacin, riboflavin, and thiamin. Instead of topping it with full-fat cream cheese, try cottage cheese or part-skim ricotta.

Banana. Widely recognized as a good source of potassium, bananas are also surprisingly rich in vitamin B_6. One 4-ounce fruit contains about 0.7 milligram of B_6, or 35 percent of the DV.

Bran muffin. A tasty way to boost your fiber intake: One $1\frac{1}{2}$-ounce muffin provides 3 grams of the nutrient. You also take in 1.8 milligrams of iron, which is about 10 percent of the DV.

Broccoli. You get over half a full day's supply of vitamin C—41 milligrams—in $\frac{1}{2}$ cup of chopped, raw broccoli. This nutrient-rich veggie offers some folate and a good amount of vitamin A, too. Eat it with low-fat dip.

cereals, cans of low-sodium vegetable juice cocktail, and whole-wheat hard pretzels.

Learn to love leftovers. "Leftovers make great snacks, provided they aren't loaded with fat," says Harper. What you choose ultimately depends on what's in your refrigerator. But don't overlook leftover pasta, cold pizza made with low-fat cheese, half a tuna

Cantaloupe. Another stellar vitamin C source: One cup of cubed cantaloupe provides 68 milligrams of C, or more than 100 percent of the DV.

Carrot. Eat a single medium-size carrot, and you'll more than satisfy your vitamin A needs for an entire day. Just one contains 17,158 international units of A, which is close to $3\frac{1}{2}$ times the DV.

Mexican-style beans. A $\frac{1}{2}$-cup serving of this filling, flavorful fare provides an impressive 7 grams of fiber—about 26 percent of the DV. Just be sure that the brand you buy doesn't go overboard on sodium.

String cheese. This lower-fat variation on mozzarella cheese supplies 250 milligrams of calcium per $1\frac{1}{2}$-ounce serving. That's about 25 percent of the DV.

Tuna. Three ounces of tuna, canned in water, is an excellent source for your daily requirement for vitamin B_{12}. You'll get 2 micrograms of the nutrient, or 32 percent of the DV. If you need to add mayonnaise, make sure it's low-fat.

Yogurt. Here's another top-notch source of bone-building calcium, with 415 milligrams—about 42 percent of the DV—in every 1-cup serving. Be sure to choose nonfat or low-fat varieties.

sandwich, or that three-bean salad you didn't have room for at lunch.

Don't retreat from treats. "Some snacks can be just for fun," says Dr. Denke. If you have a hankering for a cupcake or chips, dig in. Just be sure to compensate by choosing leaner foods for the rest of the day.

Just Desserts

Indulgence without the Guilt

BRAIN: "Strawberries."

    TASTEBUDS: "In a pie crust, buried under whipped cream."

BRAIN: "Banana."

TASTEBUDS: "Hugging three scoops of ice cream, smothered with syrup and nuts."

The great dessert debate. You want to make a healthful choice—and nutrition-wise, nothing beats fresh fruit as an after-dinner treat. But you can't ignore your tastebuds' contention that fruit alone is not dessert.

No, indeed, it's not. So indulge. There are a couple of reasons why you should. First, when you deny yourself food that you really want, you eventually stuff yourself with much more of it once you finally cave in. Second, the sweetness of dessert signals your brain that feeding time has officially ended. You feel satisfied, so you won't spend your evening browsing your kitchen for munchies.

Besides, if you're going to eat a sweet, it's best that you tack it on to a meal, says Nancy Clark, R.D., director of nutrition services at SportsMedicine Brookline in Brookline, Massachusetts, and author of *Nancy Clark's Sports Nutrition Guidebook*. That way, the fiber, protein, and tiny amount of fat in the other foods can slow the absorption of sugar into your blood-stream. Your blood sugar level holds steady, which in turn keeps your energy supply on a more even keel.

Happy Endings

While dessert has its place in a healthy diet, you do need to exercise some restraint. Cheesecake, hot fudge sundaes, and other high-fat goodies are once-a-week fare, at most. When you do feel the urge to splurge, here's how to do it right.

Make the most of every mouthful. Eat *sloooowly,* allowing every bite to linger on your tongue.

It takes a while for your brain to acknowledge the fact that you're having dessert. Relax your pace, and you will have eaten less by the time your brain gets the message and calls off your craving for a sweet.

Stay single. Stick with individually wrapped goodies. "It's better to buy a box of Fudgsicles than ½ gallon of ice cream," says Georgia Kostas, R.D., director of nutrition at the Cooper Clinic in Dallas and author of *The Balancing Act Nutrition and Weight Guide*. "That gives you built-in portion control."

Spot the sneaky treats. Some desserts taste like they have much more fat than they actually do. Among them are angel food cake (0.1 gram of fat per serving), fig bars (1 gram), fortune cookies (0 gram), ladyfingers (2 grams), and rice pudding (4 grams). Any of these can satisfy your sweet tooth without guilt.

Grab your toothbrush. Once you've swallowed your last bite, brush your teeth right away. No, you're not trying to get rid of the evidence. Like eating the dessert itself, brushing sends your brain the message that you're finished eating—and that can switch off late-night cravings.

Top 50 Low-Fat Foods

Tastes You're Bound to Love

Beethoven or the Beatles. Pinstripes or polka dots. Ballet or baseball.

So much in life is a matter of taste—especially what you eat. Regardless of how wholesome a food is, if it doesn't please your palate, it will never make it past your bicuspids without throwing your tongue into turmoil.

But good taste and good nutrition don't have to be mutually exclusive. These days we have more eating options than ever, from the growing assortment of exotic fruits and vegetables in the supermarket produce aisle to the expanded selection of packaged nonfat and low-fat products. Thanks to modern technology, junk foods have become healthier, and health foods have undergone a flavor face-lift.

So when it comes to making choices from the vast new assortment of low-fat flavors, what appeals most deliciously to our tastebuds?

To find out, we conducted an informal survey of 100 health-conscious people to get their vote on the most flavorful low-fat foods. Then, just to make sure these low-fat faves actually are low in fat and good for you, we ran the list by Toni Ferrang, R.D., owner of

Food for Thought Nutrition Consulting in Burlingame, California.

Here, then, are the top 50 low-fat foods, rated by a random sampling of Americans and arranged from A to Z.

1. Angel food cake. "Great!" Ferrang says. "Make it even better by topping it with cut-up fruit and some nonfat or low-fat yogurt."

2. Apples. Our survey takers love apples for their crunch and portability. They're a good source of fiber, too, Ferrang notes.

3. Bagels. "The best low-fat food God ever made," one respondent raves.

"Just keep in mind that a typical bagel-shop bagel has 200 to 350 calories," Ferrang says. "You'd be better off eating half of one with some fruit."

4. Baked potato chips. Based on our respondents' experiences, baked potato chips taste better than previous attempts at low-fat potato chips, and they aren't as greasy as regular chips. Even better, Ferrang adds, some brands have only 1 gram of fat per serving.

5. Baked potatoes. "To get the fiber, eat the skin," Ferrang says.

6. Bananas. "A banana is the easiest thing in the world to stick in your bag and carry to work or wherever," one person observes.

7. Beans. These fiber-rich legumes win kudos for their versatility. "And they seem to give you substance without weight," noted another person.

8. Berries. Blueberries, raspberries, and strawberries are all low-calorie and practically nonfat, and they're loaded with vitamins and minerals to boot,

Ferrang says. One respondent likes to eat fresh berries that are semifrozen—"kind of like Popsicle bites," she explains.

9. Brownies. The low-fat kind, of course. "If you combine a low-fat brownie with a piece of fruit, you have a good snack," says Ferrang.

10. Cantaloupe. This sweet-tasting fruit makes summertime low-fat eating a breeze. "It's loaded with beta-carotene," Ferrang notes.

11. Carrots. Many people like to keep carrots handy—washed, cut up, and ready to eat.

12. Cereals. "I love cereals because they're really crunchy and I can get the sweetness I like," offers one person. She thinks Cheerios leads the pack for flavor.

13. Chocolate syrup. For chocoholics, nothing beats chocolate syrup since it has plenty of flavor but no fat. Ferrang recommends mixing it in skim or low-fat (1 percent) milk for a healthy treat.

14. Corn on the cob. "A great choice," comments Ferrang. One person recommends seasoning it with spices instead of the usual butter and salt.

15. Cottage cheese. Many people have ingenious ways of enjoying this old diet staple. One suggests adding herbs such as chives for a super-easy dip or spread. Another adds it to tomato soup for an interesting mix of flavors.

16. Couscous. "Serve this grain with veggies—lots of veggies—for a more nutritionally rounded meal," Ferrang suggests.

17. Crackers. Be very careful with crackers, Ferrang says. "You can easily eat the calorie equivalent of three or four slices of toast." Be sure to choose a nonfat or low-fat version, she adds.

18. Cupcakes. The low-fat varieties can cure a craving for sweets quite nicely, our survey takers say. "But be aware that you're getting virtually no nutritional value for the calories you're consuming," Ferrang cautions.

19. Fig or fruit bars. Great to satisfy a sweet tooth.

20. Frozen yogurt. No food evokes as much passion as this one. Women rhapsodize about their favorite brands and flavors, from nonfat peach to low-fat Death by Chocolate. And all agree that it tastes even better than ice cream. However, frozen yogurt doesn't supply the amount of calcium that regular yogurt does, Ferrang says.

21. Graham crackers. Just like "regular" crackers, you can overdo with graham crackers quite easily, Ferrang notes. Still, she says, they're better than cookies.

22. Grapefruit. "I love the tart, fresh flavor of a grapefruit—even though peeling one sometimes takes a while," one respondent writes. It's worth the time, Ferrang replies, since the fruit is so rich in vitamin C.

23. Grapes. They taste great frozen, noted several people.

24. Hot chocolate. "I make mine with skim milk," one respondent says. "It turns out really creamy, and it's a great chocolate fix." Choose a nonfat, sugar-free mix to save calories, Ferrang suggests.

25. Ice cream. Nonfat and low-fat varieties of ice cream hold their own against the real thing, people agree. Ferrang says to try topping it with fruit to make it more nutrient-dense—and to keep you from going for a second serving.

26. Italian ice. Sweet and refreshing—a perfect summertime treat, respondents say. But watch the sugar content, Ferrang advises.

27. Licorice. A number of respondents applaud the chewy texture of this low-fat sweet. But licorice also packs a hefty amount of sugar, Ferrang warns.

28. Mixed greens. Many supermarkets now carry ready-to-eat mixed greens that have already been washed and cut up. "They make preparing a salad so much more convenient," one person points out. Dress up your greens healthfully with lemon juice, balsamic vinegar, and a dash of soy sauce, Ferrang suggests.

29. Oatmeal. A classic comfort food for many people. "Stick with plain oatmeal that you can season yourself," Ferrang advises. "The flavored varieties (in the packets) have a lot of sugar."

30. Oranges. This citrus superstar supplies lots of vitamins and minerals—especially vitamin C—for hardly any calories or fat, according to Ferrang.

31. Pasta. Ferrang says your best bet is to downsize the portion of pasta and add lots of veggies.

32. Pears. One person describes them as "low-fat art."

33. Peppermint patties. "You get the satisfaction of eating chocolate without overindulgence," says one person. And they come in minis, which is the perfect serving size. Mini patties are a good idea because, like any candy, patties are loaded with sugar, Ferrang says.

34. Peppers. Votes for this veggie ran the gamut from fresh bell peppers to spicy pickled peppers. It's the crunch factor that seems to win over people. And as Ferrang points out, peppers have lots of vitamin C, too.

35. Pickles. "I like to eat garlic dill pickles when I get home from work," one woman says. "They don't spoil my appetite for dinner, and they have just a few calories."

36. Popcorn. This snack gets great accolades. Most go for the air-popped kind, though some favor low-fat microwavable varieties. Popcorn is higher in fiber than most snacks, Ferrang adds. You can flavor it with spices or with nonfat butter spray.

37. Pretzels. For many people, pretzels defuse cravings by delivering a one-two punch of salt and crunch. Most have no fat, Ferrang adds, and you can get them without salt, which really is better for you.

38. Prunes. "Prunes satisfy my craving for sweets," one respondent notes. "They're filling without being fattening, and they give me an energy boost, too."

39. Pudding. Chocolate pudding made with skim milk, to be exact. Ferrang suggests opting for the sugar-free mix to save on calories.

40. Raisins. Munch on these for healthy doses of fiber, iron, and vitamin C, Ferrang says. Your sweet tooth will get a quick fix, too.

41. Refried beans. The low-fat or nonfat kind, of course. "They're just as spicy and filling and satisfying as the lard-laden kind," one person points out.

42. Skim milk. A great way to get your calcium. If you shy away from skim, try it with a shot of chocolate syrup.

43. Sorbet. "I've successfully turned my deep need for ice cream into a sorbet fetish," one person writes. Sorbet is a good alternative to full-fat ice cream, but keep an eye on those calories from sugar, Ferrang advises.

44. Strawberries. For a real treat, buy them in season and add them to low-fat cereal with skim milk.

45. Sweet potatoes. "I really like sweet potatoes because they're so sweet and yummy just plain—without adding all kinds of butter, salt, and other bad things," one person writes. If you want, Ferrang says, you can add a little honey or orange juice for flavor.

46. Tomatoes. "In the summer, you can eat them just like an apple," says one person. And they're packed with vitamin C, Ferrang says. Sprinkle tomato slices with fresh basil and pepper, then add a splash of olive oil or even a little feta cheese.

47. Tortilla chips with homemade salsa. "Wonderful, as long as the chips are baked," Ferrang says. "Add chopped peppers, onions, and mushrooms for extra flavor." The veggies provide bulk, too, so you'll feel full on fewer chips.

48. Watermelon. "It's refreshing and thirst-quenching—food and drink all in one," according to one respondent.

49. Whipped topping. Several survey takers nominate whipped topping as the best medicine for an aching sweet tooth. If you must eat it, stick with the nonfat version, Ferrang advises.

50. Yogurt. Our survey-takers express strong brand loyalty here. But overall, it's the creamy texture of nonfat and low-fat yogurt that appeals to their taste-buds. You can add some fiber to this healthy treat by slicing some fruit on top, Ferrang suggests. Other favorite toppings include cinnamon, low-fat granola, and Grape-Nuts cereal.

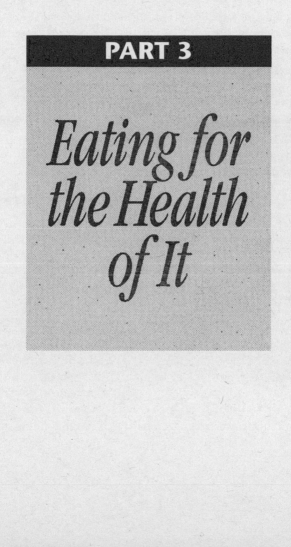

PART 3

Eating for the Health of It

Your Breast Protection

Eat the Anti-Cancer Foods

At age 30, your odds of developing breast cancer are 1 in 2,525. They climb to 1 in 93 by age 45. And by the time you're 85, they stand at 1 in 9.

Thankfully, advances in both detection and treatment have dramatically improved the breast cancer survival rate. But given a choice between surviving the disease and preventing it, wouldn't you prefer the latter?

Granted, some risk factors you can't control, such as genetics and family history. But they account for a mere fraction of all breast cancer cases. Even if they do apply to you, that doesn't mean cancer is inevitable. But there is one risk factor you can do something about: your eating habits.

Weighing the Evidence

Scientists have yet to isolate the cause—or causes—of breast cancer. But they have firmly established a link between diet and the disease. Much of their work has centered on women in Asian countries such as China and Japan, where breast cancer rates are four to seven times lower than in the United States.

Interestingly, when Asian women come to live in this country, their breast cancer risk doubles in just 10 years, according to nutritional epidemiologist Regina Ziegler, Ph.D., of the National Cancer Institute. And as generations pass, the women's risk eventually catches up with that of the "native" population.

What causes their breast cancer rates to skyrocket? Dietary changes are at least partly to blame, Dr. Ziegler says. The women start eating a lot more meat—and, consequently, more fat—while cutting back on vegetables, grains, and soy, the healthy staples of Asian cuisine.

Dietary fat promotes breast cancer in two ways. First, a high-fat diet causes your body to produce more free radicals, renegade molecules that not only damage healthy cells but also increase damage to the cell's genetic material. The greater the amount of damage, the greater the odds of developing tumors.

Second, dietary fat easily converts to body fat. And body fat, in turn, churns out the hormone estrogen. Normally, estrogen acts as a reproductive regulator, maintaining the menstrual cycle and supporting fertility. But when too much of the hormone floats around your system, it can prompt breast cells to multiply, mutate, and form cancerous breast tumors.

Your Bosom Buddies

Within the medical community, not everyone agrees on the extent to which dietary fat influences the development of breast cancer. But even those who favor a "wait and see" approach to the issue generally regard a well-balanced, low-fat diet with plenty of fruits, vegetables, and whole grains as one of the best things you can do for your overall health.

And guess what? If you follow the dietary guidelines presented in the *Prevention* Food Pyramid for Women (see page 43), you'll give yourself a big head start in the battle against breast cancer. You can make your eating habits even more breast-friendly by trying these tips from the experts.

Go easy on alcohol. In a major study on the alcohol–breast cancer link, researchers concluded that a woman who averages one drink a day over a lifetime could increase her breast cancer risk by 30 to 40 percent. Up the ante to two drinks a day, and her risk could grow by almost 70 percent.

Alcohol of any kind appears to increase the amount of estrogen circulating in the body. So if you do imbibe, try to limit yourself to just two or three drinks a week, advises JoAnn E. Manson, M.D., associate professor of medicine at Harvard Medical School and co-director of women's health at Brigham and Women's Hospital in Boston. (A drink is defined as 5 ounces of wine, 12 ounces of regular beer, or a mixed drink made with 1½ ounces of 80-proof distilled spirits.)

What about reports that a drink a day can protect you from heart attacks? "If you don't have risk factors for heart disease, then the benefit from alcohol consumption is small, and in younger women is outweighed by the higher risk of breast cancer," says Dr. Manson.

Aim low. Some experts recommend that you get no more than 25 percent of your calories from fat. Other experts say that you would boost the benefit to your breasts by knocking the fat content down a few more notches—to, say, 20 percent of calories. As a bonus, at least one study has found that this lower fat intake can help to relieve painful breasts.

Favor fiber. Fiber should be part of every woman's anti–breast cancer arsenal, according to nutrition researcher Jean H. Hankin, R.D., Dr.P.H., of the etiology program of the Cancer Research Center of

Banish Caffeine—And Breast Pain

For 4 years, Dorothy Walker, a publishing consultant in Whitehall, Pennsylvania, tolerated excruciating breast pain—until she cut out caffeine and returned to a practically pain-free life. Here's her story.

I dealt with breast pain for years—that on-and-off aching feeling that many women experience during their menstrual cycles. At age 33, however, the pain became chronic: Any accidental brush against my breasts made me cringe; taking a shower and lying in bed were painful. I tried over-the-counter pain relievers, but nothing worked.

When my breasts became increasingly hard, my doctor removed two benign fibroid cysts, but the pain continued.

Then I read a magazine article touting the pain-relieving benefits of avoiding caffeine. I immediately eliminated all caffeine from my diet—cold turkey. In retrospect, I realize that I should have gradually tapered off from my heavy caffeine intake because I went through extreme withdrawal. The severe symptoms lasted a couple of months, and it took almost a year to ride out the remaining symptoms.

The results have made it all worthwhile. Many of the cysts have disappeared, and the ones that remain are much smaller. I have a spot on my left breast that is sometimes sore, but other than that, the pain is gone. The difference is incredible!

Hawaii and professor of public health at the University of Hawaii in Honolulu. Scientists believe that fiber may reduce breast cancer risk by binding with excess estrogen and ushering it out of the body before it has a chance to do harm. Fiber also appears to interfere with the absorption of dietary fat, which, as you'll recall, ultimately serves as a catalyst for estrogen production.

The National Cancer Institute recommends an intake of 20 to 30 grams of fiber a day. You can hit the mark by eating lots of whole grains, beans, fruits, and vegetables.

Crunch crucifers. Time and again, research has shown that women who eat lots of fruits and vegetables are much less likely to develop breast cancer than women who don't. Among the best cancer-fighters in the supermarket produce aisle are the crucifers—broccoli, Brussels sprouts, cabbage, and cauliflower. These veggies contain a number of compounds, called phytochemicals, that put the squeeze on estrogen and prevent it from becoming destructive.

To preserve their phyto punch, eat crucifers raw. If you don't like them that way, then cook them until they're just tender. Canadian researchers have found that prolonged cooking can reduce the amount of at least one of the cancer-combating compounds in crucifers by as much as 50 percent.

Go fishin'. Fish such as Atlantic herring, canned pink salmon, and bluefin tuna are rich in omega-3 fatty acids. Laboratory evidence suggests that these fatty acids can stymie the growth of cancerous breast tissue.

Gobble garlic. Researchers at Memorial Sloan-Kettering Cancer Center in New York City have isolated four compounds in garlic that appear to stop breast cells from becoming cancerous in laboratory tests. These compounds also help to convert estrogen to a weaker form that isn't as likely to instigate breast cancer.

Savor soy foods. Soy is a staple in many Asian countries, and researchers believe that it's responsible for keeping the breast cancer rates among Asian women so low. It contains isoflavones, phytochemicals that mimic the hormone estrogen in the body but are 100,000 times weaker than the real thing. The isoflavones occupy places on breast cells called receptor sites, blocking estrogen from doing so.

The average Asian consumes 50 or more milligrams of soy isoflavones daily. But research suggests that if you eat just one serving of soy, that may be enough for you to experience some of its protective effects. Try adding cooked soybeans to chili, stir-frying tofu in place of meat for a variety of dishes, or drinking soy milk, which can be found in health food stores and some grocery stores. Keep in mind, however, that soy sauce and soybean oil don't contain isoflavones.

Favor flaxseed. Flaxseed contains compounds called lignan precursors. Scientists have just begun investigating how these phytochemicals work. Early studies show that lignan precursors change into a weak form of estrogen in the body and then act pretty much like isoflavones.

Try sprinkling 2 heaping tablespoons (about 25 grams) of ground flaxseed on cereal or in juice. Check your favorite health food store or baking catalog to find flaxseed.

Opt for olive oil. In a study involving more than 2,000 Greek women, those who consumed olive oil at least once a day were 25 percent less likely to develop breast cancer than those who didn't. Scientists can't yet explain how the oil protects against cancer, but they believe it has something to do with antioxidants in the oil.

Lean toward E. Vitamin E flexes its cancer-fighting muscle in several ways. First, it's an antioxidant, which means it helps mop up those damaging free radicals and prevents them from doing harm. Second, it keeps your immune system in good working order. And third, it appears to thwart the formation of cancer-causing compounds in your body.

One of the best sources of Vitamin E is wheat germ: A serving of 1⅔ tablespoons contains 4 international units of E. You'll also find the vitamin in vegetable oils, including olive oil. Just make sure that the oil you choose has mostly unsaturated fat.

The Heart Facts

Foods to Reduce Risk

Heart disease has long had a reputation as a strictly male malady. True, it tends to affect men earlier in life—women get about a 10-year grace period. But once women reach menopause, any female advantage quickly dissipates. In fact, 11 times as many women die from heart disease as from breast cancer, earning it the dubious distinction as the number one cause of death among adult women in the United States.

And man or woman, you're at greater risk of

heart disease if there are other health and lifestyle concerns in your life. What sorts of things are we talking about? For one, family history. A parent diagnosed with heart disease before age 60 puts you at higher risk of heart disease. Other factors: diabetes, high blood pressure, high cholesterol, overweight, physical inactivity, smoking, and high levels of stress—and not necessarily in that order. Each of these is a serious concern in and of itself, and your overall risk of heart problems only climbs as the risk factors add up.

None of these factors, however, is a guarantee that you're going to develop heart disease in your lifetime. In fact, every one can be offset to some degree simply by eating right.

How to Avoid a Broken Heart

What qualifies as "eating right"? Doctors say it's a combination of cutting your fat intake and filling up on fruits, vegetables, and fiber-rich grains and beans. Let's take a closer look at each of these heart-healthy nutrition strategies.

Skimp on fat. Most doctors recommend that you limit your fat intake to about 25 percent of calories— much less than the 34 percent of calories that the average American consumes. And most of that fat should be unsaturated, suggests Alice Lichtenstein, D.Sc., associate professor and research scientist at the Jean Mayer USDA Human Nutrition Research Center on Aging at Tufts University in Boston. The reason is that both monounsaturated fat (found in olive and canola oils and most nuts) and polyunsaturated fat (found in corn, safflower, and sunflower oils) actually support heart health by reducing LDL cholesterol while leaving

HDL cholesterol unchanged. That's important because your body needs HDL to flush out LDL.

On the other hand, saturated fat, found mainly in animal foods, increases heart disease risk. The link between the two is so strong that the American Heart Association recommends getting no more (and preferably less) than 10 percent of your calories from saturated fat.

Feast on fiber. Fiber—especially the soluble kind found in grains, beans, and fruits—binds with cholesterol in the body and helps remove it along with the waste, explains Diane Grabowski-Nepa, R.D., nutritional counselor at the Pritikin Longevity Center in Malibu, California. Researchers cannot yet explain how fiber works its cholesterol-clobbering magic. One popular theory is that it binds with bile acids in the intestines and escorts these cholesterol-laden compounds from your body. Your body then has to recruit more cholesterol to make more bile acids, reducing your blood cholesterol level in the process.

How much fiber does it take to safeguard your health? Between 20 and 30 grams a day, according to the National Cancer Institute.

Add some antioxidants. Vitamins C and E and beta-carotene are antioxidants. As their name suggests, the antioxidants protect against oxidation, a naturally occurring process in which renegade oxygen molecules called free radicals damage healthy cells and contribute to the artery-clogging process.

Just how protective are these nutrients? When researchers at Harvard University compared the diets of more than 87,000 nurses, they found that the nurses who ate the most antioxidant-rich foods were 46 percent less likely to develop heart disease than the nurses who ate the least.

At the very least, experts say, you should make sure that you're getting the Daily Values (DVs) of vitamins C and E—60 milligrams and 30 international units (IU), respectively. No DV has been established for beta-carotene—but you need a daily intake of about 5,000 IU to match the DV of vitamin A. (Your body converts beta-carotene to vitamin A.)

A Plateful of Prevention

To help you get in the swing of heart-smart eating, we've come up with a list of foods that meet all three of the criteria outlined above. Most have less than 1 gram of fat, the two exceptions being chickpeas and wheat germ (which, incidentally, are still considered low-fat). Each one is high in fiber. All supply healthy doses of one or more of the antioxidants. And as a bonus, not one of these foods has even a smidgen of dietary cholesterol.

Apples. One medium-size fruit (about 5 ounces) has 3 grams of fiber, 8 milligrams of vitamin C, and 0.6 IU of vitamin E.

Apricots. You get 111 milligrams of vitamin C—almost two times the DV—in three fresh apricots. They also provide 2 grams of fiber and 1 IU of beta-carotene.

Blackberries. One cup of berries contains 30 milligrams of vitamin C, along with 7 grams of fiber and 0.1 IU of vitamin E.

Black currants. One cup of black currants meets the DV of vitamin C more than three times over, supplying 203 milligrams of the nutrient. You also get 4 grams of fiber and 0.7 IU of vitamin E.

Broccoli. One-half cup of cooked chopped broccoli offers almost a whole day's worth of vitamin C: 58 milligrams. The same-size serving also contains 2 grams of fiber and 0.3 IU of beta-carotene.

Brussels sprouts. You get 3 grams of fiber, 48 grams of vitamin C, and 0.2 IU of beta-carotene in ½ cup of boiled brussels sprouts.

Butternut squash. One-half cup of baked cubed butternut squash provides 16 IU of beta-carotene. It also provides good amounts of fiber (3 grams) and vitamin C (15 milligrams).

Cantaloupe. Chow down on cantaloupe, and you can cover your vitamin C needs for an entire day. A 1-cup serving of cubed fruit supplies 68 milligrams of vitamin C as well as 1 gram of fiber and 16 IU of beta-carotene.

Carrots. One of the best vitamin A sources around: One 2½-ounce carrot has 6,745 IU of the nutrient—all you need for an entire day. You also get a nice amount of fiber (2 grams) and even a little bit of vitamin C (7 milligrams).

Chickpeas. You get a whopping 7 grams of fiber in ½ cup of chickpeas—noteworthy even for a member of the fiber-rich legume clan. The same size serving also offers a small burst of vitamin C (5 milligrams).

Grapefruit. Both pink and red varieties provide 50 milligrams of vitamin C as well as 0.7 gram of fiber.

Green peas. You can bump up your fiber intake a notch or two with these legumes. A ½-cup serving of boiled green peas offers a modest 2 grams of fiber, along with 11 milligrams of vitamin C.

Papaya. Yet another superb source of vitamin C: Half of a papaya supplies 94 milligrams of C—roughly 1½ times the DV. It also has a respectable 3 grams of fiber.

Passion fruit. It seems fitting that a food named "passion fruit" can do so much for your heart!

A serving of five medium-size fruits (about 3½ ounces total) provides decent amounts of fiber (2 grams), vitamin C (30 milligrams), and beta-carotene (0.2 IU).

Raspberries. One cup of berries gives you a hefty 6 grams of fiber as well as 31 milligrams of vitamin C.

Spinach. For beta-carotene, spinach is one of your best bets. A ½-cup serving of boiled spinach provides 25 IU of beta-carotene as well as 2 grams of fiber and 9 milligrams of vitamin C.

Strawberries. These bountiful berries offer 85 milligrams of vitamin C and 4 grams of fiber in every 1-cup serving.

Sweet potatoes. Sweet potatoes pack a beta-carotene punch, with one baked 4-ounce spud supplying 83 IU of the nutrient. As a bonus, it can boost your intake of fiber (3 grams) and vitamin C (28 milligrams).

Sweet red peppers. One-half cup of chopped red peppers has only 0.8 gram of fiber and 1 IU of beta-carotene. But you get more than a day's supply of vitamin C—95 milligrams.

Wheat germ. One-quarter cup of toasted wheat germ contains 3 IU of vitamin E, making the grain one of the best food sources of E. You get a good 4 grams of fiber, too.

Boning Up

Call In the Calcium Troops

A woman bumps into her kitchen table and shatters her hip. Seem far-fetched? About 240,000 women a year can tell you otherwise. They probably never would have believed such a minor incident could cause such a catastrophic injury—until it happened to them.

They're just a relative handful of the more than 22.4 *million* Americans who face the threats of osteoporosis, a disease that weakens the bones and leaves them vulnerable to breaking. It's responsible for an estimated 1.5 million fractures every year—mostly of the hip, wrist, and spine.

While osteoporosis affects both sexes, it seems to target women with particular ferocity. By one estimate, as many as one in two women is going to experience an osteoporosis-related fracture, compared with one in five men.

But there is a bright spot among these bleak statistics. Osteoporosis doesn't happen overnight. It takes a lifetime to develop. So if you act now, you can help protect your skeleton from this insidious disease.

The best prescription for your bone health? Engage in weight-bearing exercise (such as walking, running, or aerobics), give up smoking (if you do), and—perhaps most important—eat lots of bone-friendly foods. In fact, one estimate suggests that the right diet alone could prevent as many as half of all osteoporosis-related fractures.

Growing, Growing—Gone

To understand how osteoporosis works, you should first know a little bit about the bone-building process itself. Throughout your life, your body constantly removes old bone tissue and replaces it with fresh stuff. The gains surpass the losses until sometime in your

Do You Fit This M.O.?

The National Osteoporosis Foundation has put together the following osteoporosis risk assessment for women. Keep in mind that a "yes" response to any question doesn't mean that osteoporosis is inevitable. You just have to take some extra precautions to protect your bone density.

1. Do you have a small, thin frame?
2. Are you Caucasian or Asian?
3. Do you have a family history of osteoporosis?
4. Have you been through menopause?
5. Have you had an early or a surgically induced menopause?
6. Have you been taking thyroid medication or high doses of cortisone-like drugs for asthma, arthritis, or cancer?
7. Is your diet low in calcium?
8. Are you physically inactive?
9. Do you smoke cigarettes or drink alcohol in excess?

thirties, when you reach what is called your peak bone mass. Then your body institutes its own version of downsizing: It continues to get rid of old bone tissue, but it doesn't bother to fill all the vacancies. Demand exceeds supply, and you end up losing about 1 percent of your bone mass every year.

This rate of bone loss is considered normal. Everyone experiences it—women as well as men. But in osteoporosis, some additional factor kicks bone loss into overdrive. For women, that additional factor is usually menopause.

Up until menopause, a woman's body has an abundant supply of the hormone estrogen. Estrogen helps to keep the skeleton healthy and strong. So when estrogen production declines at menopause, bone density does, too. In the 5 to 7 years following menopause, a woman can lose 2 to 3 percent of her bone mass a year—or up to about 20 percent.

While it's true that you can't replace lost bone, you can do a lot to preserve the bone you have. You can start by reinforcing your diet with calcium, your best ally in the battle against bone loss.

In This Corner: Calcium

To show you just how important calcium is, in 1994 the National Institutes of Health convened a special panel to set optimum intake guidelines for women and men of all ages. Here's a quick recap of the panel's recommendations for women.

♦ Ages 25 to 50: 1,000 milligrams

♦ Ages 51 to 65 (postmenopausal) and taking hormone replacement therapy: 1,000 milligrams

♦ Ages 51 to 65 (postmenopausal) and not taking hormone replacement therapy: 1,500 milligrams

♦ Age 66 plus: 1,500 milligrams

♦ Pregnant or nursing: 1,200 to 1,500 milligrams

Unfortunately, most American women aren't hitting the 1,000-milligram mark—not by a long shot. The average intake is a paltry 450 milligrams a day. Why? Part of the problem, suggests Susan Broy, M.D., director of the Osteoporosis Center at the Advocate Medical Group in Chicago, is that women have forsaken some of the best food sources of calcium—namely, dairy products such as milk and cheese—because of their high fat content. It may very well be that in trying to protect her heart and waistline from fat's follies, the average woman is putting her bones at risk.

Befriend the Bone-Builders

By no means are we suggesting that you feast on high-fat fare for your bones' sake. Experts say that there are plenty of healthy ways that you can meet your daily calcium quota through diet.

The following nutrition strategies can keep your bone bank in the black—and save your skeleton for a lifetime.

Rediscover dairy. Have you paid a visit to your supermarket's dairy case lately? If not, you should. You'll find an almost mind-boggling array of nonfat and low-fat dairy products, including milk, cheese, and yogurt. And just because the fat is gone doesn't mean the calcium is, Dr. Broy notes. For example, an 8-ounce glass of skim milk contains 300 milligrams of calcium. Drink 3½ glasses a day, and you'll get all of the mineral you need.

Graze on greens. They don't supply as much calcium as dairy products do, but dark green, leafy vegetables can definitely move you a few rungs up the ladder to your recommended daily intake. Among the calcium standouts in this produce group are kale, with 47 milligrams per ½ cup, and broccoli, with 36 milligrams per ½ cup.

Grow fond of fish. Certain fish have edible bones that are loaded with calcium. For example, 3 ounces of canned pink salmon has 181 milligrams of the mineral, while 1 ounce of canned Atlantic sardines has 92 milligrams. Canned fish does have a lot of sodium, though, so look for brands labeled "low-salt" and, in the case of sardines, rinse them well before eating.

Seek out surprise sources. Many manufacturers now add calcium to certain packaged foods. Calcium-fortified orange juice, for instance, supplies just as much of the mineral as skim milk: 300 milligrams in an 8-ounce glass.

Nosh at night. As mentioned earlier, your body is constantly dumping old bone tissue. But at least one study has shown that the process actually speeds up while you sleep, peaking at about 3:00 A.M. Having a calcium-rich nightcap—maybe a glass of skim milk or some nonfat yogurt—may keep your blood level of the mineral more stable during the overnight hours.

Don't forget D. Calcium can't do its job without vitamin D to escort it across intestinal walls and into your bone cells. Your body can manufacture its own D with a little help from the sun. But if you live in a northern climate or don't spend 5 to 15 minutes in direct sunlight without sunscreen every day, you'll want to make sure that you're getting enough of the nutrient from food sources instead. Both milk and breakfast cereals are fortified with vitamin D. Aim for the Daily Value (DV) of 400 IU.

Watch your tempeh. Tempeh, tofu, and other soy foods contain estrogen-like compounds called isoflavones. Scientists at the University of Illinois found that women who consumed 90 milligrams of iso-flavones a day experienced a 2 percent increase in their bone densities. You can reach 90 milligrams—the amount used in the study—by eating 1 cup of roasted soy nuts (60 milligrams) and drinking 1 cup of soy milk (30 milligrams).

By the way, not all soy foods contain isoflavones. You won't find them in soy sauce or soybean oil, for example.

Beware the Bone-Robbers

Just as some foods can safeguard your skeletal strength, others seem to steal it away. To rid your diet of the leading bone-offenders, heed this advice from the experts.

Stop the a-salt. A high-sodium diet delivers a double whammy to your skeleton. Salt not only inter-feres with calcium absorption but also increases the amount of the mineral that's excreted from your body.

You don't necessarily have to give up salt entirely, says Edith Howard Hogan, R.D., a dietitian in Washington, D.C., and a spokesperson for the American Dietetic Association. But a little moderation is in order. Ideally, experts say, you should get no more than the DV of 2,400 milligrams of salt a day—the equivalent of about 1 teaspoon.

Quaff coffee with caution. Some studies suggest that drinking a lot of coffee—or any caffeine-laden beverage, for that matter—may raise your risk of a hip fracture. Based on what they know so far, experts believe that you can have up to two cups of java a day without any ill effects.

And rather than drinking your coffee black, try adding a little milk, suggests Jeri W. Nieves, Ph.D., nutritional epidemiologist at Columbia University in New York City and director of the bone mineral measurement laboratory at Helen Hayes Hospital in West Haverstraw, New York. Milk prevents caffeine from stealing calcium from your bones.

Give cola the cold shoulder. It's not only the caffeine in cola that can be hard on your bones. Preliminary research suggests that phosphorus—a mineral found in cola as well as in many processed foods—contributes to higher rates of bone fracture.

Some scientists believe that phosphorus actually steps up calcium excretion. But others, including Mona S. Calvo, Ph.D., a member of the clinical research and review staff of the Office of Special Nutritionals at the Food and Drug Administration in Washington, D.C., suspect the real problem is that we're trading in milk for cola and running up a calcium deficit as a result. The combination of too much phosphorus and too little calcium leads to osteoporosis, she says.

Clearly, more research is necessary to flesh out the phosphorus-osteoporosis link. For now, experts recommend that you limit your cola consumption to one 12-ounce serving per day.

Put a lid on alcohol. Research has shown that people who drink more than two glasses of wine or 4 ounces of hard liquor a day have less bone mass than teetotalers of the same age and sex. Why? Well, alcohol not only has a direct toxic effect on bone cells, it also seems to take the place of calcium-rich foods in the diet.

The bottom line is that if you must imbibe, do so in moderation—no more than two or three drinks a week. (A drink is defined as 5 ounces of wine, 12 ounces of beer, or a mixed drink made with 1½ ounces of liquor.)

Clobber Cholesterol

What the Numbers Are Telling You

A generation ago, the word *cholesterol* would have had about as much meaning to the general population as *floppy disk* or *fax*.

These days, of course, most of us can recite our cholesterol readings as though they were our birth dates. We've taken heed of all the reports citing cholesterol as a leading risk factor for heart disease.

Those reports don't paint a flattering image of cholesterol—nor, for that matter, an entirely accurate one. To begin with, you can get the impression that cholesterol is all bad, when in reality, your body *needs* it to manufacture cell membranes, sex hormones, bile acids, and vitamin D. Your liver produces about 2,000 milligrams of the waxy, fatlike substance every day just for these routine tasks. You literally couldn't live without it.

The problems arise when there's too much cholesterol floating around your bloodstream. While genetics, lack of exercise, and smoking can all contribute to high cholesterol, a high-fat diet is usually to blame, says Debra R. Judelson, M.D., cardiologist in Beverly Hills and chair of the Cardiovascular Disease in Women Committee of the American Medical Women's Association.

But even then, not all cholesterol is bad. While one type, known as low-density lipoprotein (LDL) cholesterol, does most of the damage, another cholesterol, known as high-density lipoprotein (HDL), actually works to your health's advantage. And scientists now know that it's the ratio of the two rather than the total of the two that helps to determine your state of health.

The Female Advantage

LDL is the cholesterol with the bad reputation because it likes to congregate on the walls of your arteries. Eventually, the buildup can become so severe that it slows and can eventually shut down blood flow to the heart and brain, explains Penny Kris-Etherton, R.D., Ph.D., professor of nutrition at Pennsylvania State University in University Park. HDL, on the other hand, plays good cop by rounding up loitering LDL and running it out of your body.

Ideally, then, a healthy total cholesterol reading consists of a low level of LDL and a high level of HDL.

What the Numbers Mean

The next time your doctor orders a cholesterol test, insist on two things: a total cholesterol reading and a breakdown of the total into high-density lipoprotein (HDL) and low-density lipoprotein (LDL) and triglycerides. Some doctors don't like to do separate HDL, LDL, and triglyceride testing because it's costlier and more time-consuming. Finally, when the results come in, don't settle for a verdict like "your cholesterol is fine"; ask for the numbers.

Incidentally, many doctors rely on the ratio of total cholesterol to HDL cholesterol as a more accurate predictor of heart disease risk. You can figure out your own ratio: Simply divide your total cholesterol reading by your HDL reading. According to the American Heart Association, if the answer is 3.5 or less, your cholesterol profile is in great shape.

This is where women have a huge advantage, with average HDL readings 10 to 12 points higher than men's.

Why the difference? Scientists suspect it may have something to do with the female hormone estrogen. Estrogen seems to boost your HDL level while at the same time holding down your LDL level. This may explain why a woman's risk of heart disease rises so sharply at menopause, just as the body slows its production of estrogen.

But man or woman, you should have your cholesterol checked regularly, and when you do, make sure that the screening breaks out your LDL, HDL, and

According to experts, the following numbers will help you determine exactly where you stand.

Total Cholesterol (mg/dl)	HDL (mg/dl)	LDL (mg/dl)	Tri-glycerides (mg/dl)
DESIRABLE Below 200	Above 55 (60 or higher is protective)	Below 130 (100 or lower if you have heart disease)	Below 200
BORDERLINE 200–239	35-55	130–159	200–399
UNDESIRABLE 240 or higher	Below 35	160 or higher	400 or higher

triglyceride readings. (Triglycerides are a type of blood fat that, like cholesterol, appears to increase a person's risk for heart disease.) An HDL level of 55 to 60 is considered healthy for a woman, while men should have a count above 35. In both cases, the higher, the better, says Margo Denke, M.D., associate professor of internal medicine at the Center for Human Nutrition at the University of Texas Southwestern Medical Center at Dallas, a member of the American Heart Association's Nutrition Committee, and a member of the National Institutes of Health panel of experts on HDL and heart disease. For LDL, men and women should aim low: 130

or under. Levels of triglycerides and total cholesterol below 200 are considered ideal for men and women.

Conquering Cholesterol

The problem with cholesterol is that too few of us have ideal counts. If we did, heart disease would be way down. Research shows that for every 1 percent reduction in total cholesterol, the risk of heart attack drops 2 percent. For the most part, lowering your cholesterol is a simple matter of eating more of some foods and less of others.

Toss the yolks. Egg yolks and organ meats have no place in a low-cholesterol lifestyle. With 212 milligrams of cholesterol in a single large egg, it's just not worth it when you consider that we should be getting no more than 300 milligrams a day. Along with egg yolks, kidney and liver are the most notorious offenders.

Cut the fat. Some researchers believe that fat—especially saturated fat—may have more of an effect on your cholesterol level than dietary cholesterol itself. Like dietary cholesterol, saturated fat increases the amount of LDL circulating in your bloodstream, according to Mary Felando, R.D., a cardiovascular nutrition specialist in Los Angeles.

Conveniently, the foods that contain the most dietary cholesterol also contain the most saturated fat. Be especially wary of foods from animal sources, such as red meat and full-fat dairy products, especially butter.

Go for oil over butter. While saturated fat raises your cholesterol level, unsaturated fats have the opposite effect. Monounsaturated fat—the kind found in abundance in olive, canola, and peanut oils—lowers unhealthy LDL while preserving healthy HDL. Polyunsaturated fat lowers LDL, too, but at the expense of HDL. Still, experts agree, it's a better bet than saturated fat. You'll find polyunsaturated fat in corn, sunflower, and soybean oils.

Other food sources of unsaturated fats include whole grains, vegetables, avocados, olives, and legumes.

Give hydrogenation the heave-ho. Manufacturers use hydrogenation to harden vegetable oils into stick margarine and solid vegetable shortening. The process produces substances known as trans-fatty acids, which appear to not only raise LDL cholesterol but also lower HDL cholesterol.

If you prefer margarine over butter, stick with the tub or liquid variety. Also, go easy on fast foods and prepared baked goods—about 75 percent of the trans-fatty acids in the typical American diet come from sources such as these.

Have fish tonight. Fish such as salmon and tuna are rich in omega-3 fatty acids, a type of fat that appears to boost beneficial HDL cholesterol. To get the most benefit from omega-3's, try to eat a 3- to 4-ounce serving of fish twice a week, suggests Joanne Curran-Celentano, R.D., Ph.D., associate professor of nutritional sciences at the University of New Hampshire in Durham.

Fill up on fiber-rich foods. Soluble fiber—the kind found in beans, fruits, and grains such as oats, barley, and rye—dissolves in water to form a gel-like material that prevents cholesterol from being absorbed into your bloodstream, says Rosemary Newman, R.D., Ph.D., professor of foods and nutrition at Montana State University in Bozeman, who has studied fiber and its relationship to cholesterol since the early 1980s. When cholesterol isn't absorbed, it gets excreted from your body instead.

There's another kind of fiber, too—insoluble fiber, found in vegetables, cereals, and grains such as wheat. It increases bulk and speeds the movement of waste products—including cholesterol—through the intestines, Dr. Newman explains.

The American Heart Association recommends a daily fiber intake of 25 grams, which is in the range of what other health organizations recommend. About 25 percent of that amount, or roughly 6 grams, should be in the form of soluble fiber. "And it's a good idea to eat most of your fiber with the fattiest meal of the day, so it does its job most effectively," Dr. Newman says.

Make pectin your pal. Fruits such as apples, grapefruit, oranges, and bananas contain a special kind of soluble fiber called pectin. Like other soluble fiber, pectin blocks the absorption of cholesterol into the bloodstream. But it also seems to affect the enzymes in the liver that produce cholesterol. The more pectin that you eat, the smaller the amount of cholesterol made in your liver.

Serve up soy. Tofu and other soy foods contain phytoestrogens, compounds that help transport LDL cholesterol from the bloodstream to the liver, where it's broken down and excreted. Experts suggest aiming for two or three servings of soy foods a day to reap the cholesterol-clobbering benefits of phytoestrogens. One-half cup of tofu counts as a serving, as does 1 cup of soy milk.

Savor the "stinking rose." Garlic contains a compound called allicin that apparently has the ability to alter the way your body uses cholesterol. An analysis of the findings of five studies found that eating ½ to 1 clove of garlic a day can lower blood cholesterol an average of 9 percent. If you decide to give garlic a try, remember to mince or crush it before eating it. That releases more cholesterol-combating allicin.

Drink to your health—maybe. Scientists don't

yet know why, but alcohol can bolster beneficial HDL cholesterol—sometimes as much as moderate exercise can. Of course, if you're a woman, this news is tempered by the finding that even moderate alcohol consumption can increase your odds of developing breast cancer.

Research is under way to identify the component of wine that's beneficial to cholesterol to try to come up with a nonalcoholic substitute. Until then, Dr. Judelson advises that if you do choose to imbibe, keep it moderate: no more than two or three drinks a week.

No More Migraines

Foods to Avoid

Referring to a migraine as a headache is like referring to a tornado as a breeze. Yes, a headache hurts, even throbs. But a migraine bludgeons, crushes, tortures, incapacitates. If you've never had one—lucky you—imagine having your skull squeezed in a vise while someone pounds on it with a sledgehammer, and you get the idea.

Migraines are characterized by rapid changes in the blood vessels of the face, head, and neck. The word *migraine* comes from the Greek *hemikrania*—literally, "half cranium." It alludes to the fact that migraine typically affects only one side of the head. But it doesn't stop there.

Migraine pain can envelop your entire body, treating you to a smorgasbord of symptoms that includes nausea, vomiting, dizziness, tremors, and sensitivity to light and sound. The misery can endure anywhere from a few hours to more than a day.

Scientists are still trying to figure out the chain of events that takes place in the brain leading up to a full-blown migraine. They do know that any of a number of factors can get the ball rolling, including stress, poor sleeping habits, even a change in altitude or the weather. But one of the most common triggers of migraine pain is food.

Foes in the Fridge

According to one estimate, one in every five migraine episodes can be traced to something you ate. Dozens of foods contain natural or added substances that can alter your brain chemistry in such a way that blood vessels on the outside of your skull undergo chemical changes that irritate sensitive nerve endings, explains Russell W. Walker, M.D., chief of the Head Pain Program at the Barrow Neurological Institute in Phoenix.

Women seem especially vulnerable to such food triggers. Perhaps that's why women are three times as likely to suffer from migraines as men. Many doctors attribute this heightened susceptibility to the hormonal fluctuations that occur every month as part of the menstrual cycle. In fact, roughly 50 percent of migraine-prone women report that they most often experience attacks around the time of their periods.

You may be able to head off migraine pain, according to Dr. Walker, simply by avoiding foods that contain any of the following substances.

Aspartame. This artificial sweetener, which goes by the brand name NutraSweet, has caused its share of controversy. While researchers have not yet proven that it provokes migraines, people report experiencing more attacks when they eat foods and drink beverages that have aspartame as an ingredient.

Monosodium glutamate (MSG). Often used as a flavor enhancer in Chinese cuisine, MSG is also a common ingredient in lunch meats, canned and dried soups, and frozen dinners.

Nitrites. Food manufacturers use nitrites to preserve the color of cured meats, such as hot dogs, bacon, ham, and salami.

Vasoactive amines. Perhaps the best-known member of this class of food triggers is tyramine, an amino acid found mainly in strong aged cheeses, pickled herring, chicken livers, and the pods of lima beans and snow peas. Other vasoactive amines include phenylethylamine (in chocolate) and synephrine (in citrus fruits and juices), says Merle Diamond, M.D., associate director of the Diamond Headache Clinic in Chicago.

Another common migraine provocateur: alcohol. "In fact, it tops the list of foods that affect the most people with migraines," says Dr. Diamond. "It is a vasodilator, meaning that it expands blood vessels, which can trigger migraine."

Making Headway against the Pain

If you are migraine-prone, you can control the frequency and severity of your attacks by identifying and eliminating the foods that cause you problems. The best way to accomplish that is to keep a migraine diary, according to Dr. Diamond.

Each time you experience a migraine, record the date, time, and severity of the episode, along with any foods you have eaten. Also make note of any details that you think may be relevant—perhaps you're stressed, or you're taking medication. Then watch for a pattern to develop.

Once you've ferreted out the potential offenders, drop them from your diet and see if you notice a difference in how often migraine occurs and in how much it hurts. "You can prevent migraine at least 40 percent of the time just by making dietary changes," Dr. Diamond notes.

Just as some foods instigate migraine pain, other foods may actually help to prevent it. Here's what researchers know so far.

Count on carbohydrates. Eating more carbohydrate-rich foods can help boost levels of the brain chemical serotonin, which is responsible for transmitting messages from one nerve cell to another. A dip in your serotonin level can set the stage for migraine.

"There's no doubt that following a diet high in complex carbohydrates and low in fat can be very helpful for some people who experience migraines, although we don't know exactly why," Dr. Diamond says. So you may want to try stocking your diet with whole grains, beans, and fresh vegetables, all of which supply complex carbohydrates.

Note: If you have hypoglycemia, or low blood sugar, eating lots of complex carbohydrates may make your migraine attacks worse instead of better. In fact, you may be better off cutting back on complex carbs.

Bank on B$_6$. Like complex carbohydrates, vitamin B_6 helps to increase the levels of serotonin in the brain. So make sure that you're getting at least the Daily Value (DV) of B_6 for women, which is 2 milligrams. One medium baked potato supplies 0.7 milligram of the nutrient, or 35 percent of the DV.

Mind your minerals. Evidence suggests that getting enough calcium, iron, and magnesium in your diet can also help protect you against migraine attacks. Here are some of the latest findings about these minerals.

♦ Calcium. In one study, people who consumed 200 milligrams of calcium a day—just 20 percent of your recommended daily intake of 1,000 milligrams—experienced fewer migraine episodes than women who consumed less than that amount. Top food sources of the mineral include skim milk (302 milligrams per 8-ounce glass) and nonfat yogurt (452 milligrams per cup).

♦ Iron. If you run low on iron, your red blood cells can't transport oxygen the way they should. In response, your blood vessels dilate to allow more blood to flow through—and that may lead to migraine. If you're a woman, you should be getting at least the DV of iron, which is 18 milligrams. Men should stick with the RDA, which is 10 milligrams. Lean meats are your top choice, since they contain the type of iron that's highly absorbable. Three ounces of broiled top round steak, for example, supplies 2.5 milligrams of the mineral. An equal portion of roasted white turkey meat contains 1.2 milligrams.

♦ Magnesium. Research has shown that migraine-prone people often don't have enough magnesium in their brain cells. Correcting the shortfall may help protect against migraine pain. This "remedy" has proven especially effective for women who experience migraine during their periods. To meet the DV of 400 milligrams, check out the cereal aisle. Some brands supply more than 100 milligrams of magnesium per 1-ounce serving.

Quaff coffee. A jolt of java may help pull the plug on migraine pain since caffeine temporarily constricts dilated blood vessels, points out Dr. Diamond. But be careful not to overdo: Too much caffeine can actually trigger a migraine attack. She recommends that you limit yourself to two 5-ounce cups of coffee a day, which amounts to about 200 milligrams of caffeine.

Size up soy. Based on very preliminary research, a team of scientists at Yale University School of Medicine has theorized that soy foods may help head off one particular type of migraine. Soy contains compounds called isoflavones, which the researchers found can short-circuit migraine associated with a rare disorder called hereditary hemorrhagic telangiectasia. The results of their study need to be confirmed on a much larger scale. But given all the other wonderful things that soy can do for your good health, you have nothing to lose—and everything to gain—by giving it a try.

Treat your pain gingerly. From Odense University in Denmark come preliminary reports that the spice ginger may counteract prostaglandins, substances that cause blood vessels to become inflamed and therefore produce migraine pain. It's too soon to say what the therapeutic amount of ginger may be. But if you want to give it a try, make yourself a cup of ginger tea by steeping a teaspoon of the grated root in a cup of boiling water for at least 5 minutes, suggests

Dr. Walker. Sip the tea whenever you feel migraine coming on, he says.

Boost Immunity

The Favorite Cold and Flu Fighters

Wear your galoshes when it rains."
"Don't go outside with damp hair when it's cold."
"Stay out of drafts."
"Eat your vegetables."

Your mother probably gave you that advice for fending off colds and flu—and no doubt if you have kids, you've passed it on to them, too. Of course, doctors tell us that wet feet, damp hair, and drafts don't make us sick—germs do.

But increasingly, eating vegetables (and fruit, while you're at it) seems to hold up as a valid strategy for boosting immunity.

"When we don't eat well, the first thing to be compromised is our immune system," says Susanna Cunningham-Rundles, Ph.D., associate professor of immunology at New York Hospital–Cornell Medical Center in New York City.

Feed a Cold, Starve a Fever

Maybe there is something to this old wives' tale, says Susanna Cunningham-Rundles, Ph.D., associate professor of immunology at New York Hospital–Cornell Medical Center in New York City. When you come down with a fever, your immune system kicks into defense mode. It produces proteins called cytokines to protect your body from harmful invaders. These proteins also slow down your metabolic rate and make you feel like you don't want to eat, which gives your digestive system a rest and allows your body to use its resources to fight the invading infection.

On the other hand, feeding a cold can be very therapeutic because it helps to stimulate circulation. Further, by eating, you provide your immune cells with the vitamins and minerals they need to fight the cold. But be careful what you eat: Fatty, salty foods are more difficult to digest. Many people who have a cold crave soups and other hot foods, which is beneficial since a steaming bowl of soup opens airways and keeps mucus flowing. Chicken soup, a well-known home remedy, usually contains garlic and vegetables, well-known immunity boosters.

Whether you have a fever or a cold, however, drink plenty of fluids. Even if you aren't hungry, keep drinking juices high in vitamin C, a potent immunity protector.

The Defensive Lineup

Your immune system has special defense mechanisms that are constantly at work, protecting your body from bacterial infections or viral invasions that can cause colds and flu. Your skin and mucous membranes, and the secretions these membranes produce, constitute your first line of defense against foreign substances.

If a virus manages to slip past your outer barrier, it's met by the next level of defense, which works via immune cells in your bloodstream. Specifically, blood has two specialized types of white cells, or lymphocytes, called B cells and T cells.

B cells manufacture antibodies. T cells are the first to attack viruses and bacteria when they enter your body. They also manufacture interleukins, which carry signals through the immune system. Other immune cells, natural killer cells, kill infected cells and make interferon to protect healthy cells from infection.

The immune system is extremely selective, launching responses geared toward eliminating a specific invader. Your immune system also has an incredible memory. After your initial exposure to an infection, if this same infection ever returns, your immune system will recognize it immediately and issue a counterattack. In other words, you build immunity to infections encountered in the past.

Vitamins to the Rescue

Plant foods contain substances called antioxidants. These are disease-fighting compounds that keep our immune systems strong by protecting cells from harm. Of the many antioxidants found in nature, vitamins C and

E and beta-carotene are the most powerful. And getting enough of these compounds in your diet is easy if you know what foods to eat, says Lillie Grossman, R.D., Dr.P.H., professor of nutrition at California State University, Northridge. Here's what experts recommend.

Consume citrus for C. Vitamin C strengthens white blood cells, which are critical for fending off infection. It also lowers levels of histamine, a chemical released by the immune cells that can trigger runny noses.

The Daily Value (DV) for vitamin C is 60 milligrams. Many researchers agree that 200 milligrams may be the optimal amount that your body needs every day to protect against disease. Some of the best sources of vitamin C are citrus fruits; an orange, for example, has 70 milligrams. Other fruits and vegetables such as kiwi, cantaloupe, and broccoli are also good choices.

Nibble seeds, nuts, and wheat germ. Vitamin E has been found to increase levels of interferon and interleukin, two of the chemicals the immune system produces to fight infection. In a study at Tufts University in Medford, Massachusetts, researchers found that people taking 800 international units (IU) of vitamin E each day were able to increase their levels of interleukin.

Experts generally recommend 400 IU of vitamin E a day—well above the DV of 30 IU. Unfortunately, vitamin E is found mainly in nuts, seeds, and vegetable oils, which are also high in fat. But you don't have to eat nuts and seeds by the handful to reap their benefits. Just sprinkle a few almonds or sunflower seeds onto your salads to give them an extra antioxidant crunch. Wheat germ also supplies generous amounts of vitamin E, but without the fat and calories. Try adding it to cereal, baked goods, and casseroles.

Scout out beta-carotene. Beta-carotene stimulates the immune system's natural killer cells. Researchers at the University of Arizona in Tucson found that people getting 30 milligrams (about 50,000 IU) of beta-carotene a day produced more natural killer cells and immune-boosting lymphocytes than those getting less beta-carotene.

Beta-carotene is a plant pigment, so look for deep green, yellow, and orange fruits and vegetables when you're in the produce aisle. Dark, leafy vegetables like spinach, broccoli, turnips, and collard greens and bright orange and yellow vegetables like sweet potatoes and carrots are all excellent sources of beta-carotene. In fact, eating one carrot a day will provide 12 milligrams (20,000 IU) of beta-carotene, just under the recommended amount of 15 to 20 milligrams (25,000 to 33,000 IU) each day.

Munch Foods with Minerals

Vitamins aren't the only nutrients that help hold the line against infection. In various ways, minerals like zinc, copper, iron, magnesium, and selenium play a role in boosting immunity—and they're widely distributed in fresh foods. In fact, the less you rely on processed foods, the less apt you are to need mineral supplements to shore up immunity, says Dr. Grossman.

For mineral-smart eating, follow these guidelines recommended by Dr. Grossman.

Make seafood your zinc link. A deficiency in zinc can slow down your immune system's response to invaders, and it can cause a decline in the production of T cells. Studies have shown that people deficient in zinc are more prone to infection and immunity weakness.

Among food sources of zinc, oysters are tops. Six

medium-size steamed oysters supply 76 milligrams—about five times the DV of 15 milligrams. Lean meats are also good sources, as are wheat germ, green beans, and legumes such as pinto beans and black-eyed peas.

Do some ironing. Iron helps carry oxygen to cells, including your immune cells. In addition, your body produces fewer antibodies when it doesn't have enough iron, and as a result your immune defense becomes slowed and less destructive. Besides beans, good sources of iron include lean meats and steamed oysters and clams. Tofu and fortified cereals such as Cream of Wheat also supply an abundance of iron.

Serve up selenium-rich foods. Like vitamins C, E, and beta-carotene, selenium is an antioxidant. Needed in very small amounts, this trace mineral activates your body's infection-fighting cells and prevents oxidative damage to cells. The DV for selenium is 70 micrograms—the amount in half a tuna sandwich. Whole grains, fish, and shellfish provide the most selenium.

Mind your magnesium. This mineral helps your body manufacture infection-fighting white blood cells. The DV for magnesium is 400 milligrams. Magnesium is found primarily in whole grains, nuts, seeds, and a few of our finned friends such as mackerel.

Slip in some copper. As mineral deficiencies go, copper deficits are rare, since you need only 2 milligrams each day. Nevertheless, a deficiency of this essential trace mineral can lead to a low white blood cell count and, consequently, poor resistance to infections. Your best bet is to eat steamed oysters (without the butter bath), which have 3 milligrams of copper for a serving of six oysters.

Extra Energy

Foods for Get-Up-and-Go

At age 5, you stubbornly refused to take an afternoon nap. At 10, you routinely pleaded with your parents to let you stay up for "just 5 more minutes." At 20, you and your buddies would head out for a night on the town and not return home until the wee hours of the morning. In your thirties and forties, you devoted your daytime to your kids, and made up for it by doing the things you loved at night.

Well, all those years of brushing off Mr. Sandman have come back to haunt you. These days you don't defy sleep. You crave it. And even when you get enough you may feel sluggish and worn out just hours after rolling out of bed.

It may be small consolation, but you are not alone in your quest for zest. About one-quarter of all Americans—more women than men—go through their days feeling fatigued. And 2 to 3 percent have fatigue so severe that it's almost disabling.

No matter what is responsible for your malaise, poor eating habits can magnify the problem. Quite simply, when you don't feed your body properly, it doesn't have the nutrients it needs to perform at its peak.

The Food Factor

To understand how food influences your energy level, you need to know a little bit about what's going on inside your noggin—even as you're reading this sentence. The nerve cells in your brain communicate with each other with the help of substances called neurotransmitters. These chemical messengers can drastically affect energy levels and how you feel at any given moment. "We're talking about a whole symphony of brain chemicals that ebb and flow throughout the day," says Elizabeth Somer, R.D., author of *Nutrition for Women* and *Food and Mood*.

To produce these neurotransmitters, your brain needs certain nutrients from foods. What you eat influences which neurotransmitters are firing away in your brain.

Dopamine and norepinephrine are neurotransmitters associated with physical and mental vigor. Studies have shown that when people have high levels of dopamine and norepinephrine, they feel more energetic. Your brain manufactures these neurotransmitters with help from tyrosine, an amino acid found in high-protein foods such as fish, chicken, and low-fat yogurt.

Serotonin, on the other hand, makes you feel relaxed and snoozy, which is great at bedtime, but not at 2:00 P.M. To produce serotonin, your brain needs the amino acid tryptophan, abundant in high-carbohydrate foods such as potatoes, pasta, and rice.

Ideally, Somer says, you should choose foods that complement your energy peaks and valleys. For example, if you routinely crash in the afternoon, choose a lunch rich in protein—perhaps a tuna sandwich, skim milk, and fruit. "Then, when you need to wind down at the end of the day, go for the spaghetti dinner," she suggests.

You can also keep your energy on a more even keel by eating low-fat mini-meals instead of the standard three squares. When you don't eat for 3 to 4 hours at a shot, your blood sugar level drops slightly, explains Franca Alphin, R.D., nutrition director at the Duke University Diet and Fitness Center in Durham, North Carolina. Eating four or five small meals throughout the day stabilizes your blood sugar, which helps to fend off fatigue.

Edible Energizers

There's more to the energy equation than just protein and carbohydrates. Scientists have identified other key nutrients that keep your internal batteries charged. The following tips can help ensure that you're fueling your body properly, so you feel pumped up instead of pooped out.

Insist on iron. Fatigue is a classic symptom of iron-deficiency anemia. But even minor depletions of your body's iron stores can leave you feeling tired.

The Daily Value (DV) for iron is 18 milligrams for women; men, though, need less—just 10 milligrams will do. You can easily obtain either amount from foods. Among the best sources are lean meat, beans, tofu, and Cream of Wheat cereal.

Don't miss magnesium. Magnesium is a pivotal player in the energy production process. Your body needs the mineral to convert the food that you eat into fuel. To meet the DV of 400 milligrams, ply your diet with beans, tofu, wheat germ, nuts, and seeds.

Zero in on zinc. Like magnesium, zinc supports energy production and helps your pancreas manufacture the hormone insulin, which in turn boosts delivery of blood sugar—your body's basic fuel—to cells. Aim for the DV of 15 milligrams a day. Steamed oysters are an outstanding zinc source, as are wheat germ and lean beef.

B your best. A shortage of B vitamins can leave your body struggling to convert food into usable energy. The DVs for vitamin B_6 and folate are 2 milligrams and 400 micrograms, respectively. You'll find B_6 in abundant supply in bananas, cabbage, cauliflower, and wheat germ. For folate, choose beans, carrots, pumpkin, and dark green, leafy vegetables such as spinach.

Stay hydrated. Allowing yourself to run dry can sap your stamina and leave you feeling sluggish. Try to drink at least eight 8-ounce glasses of water a day.

Don't Let Them Fuel You

Many of the foods we normally turn to for a quick pick-me-up actually end up letting us down instead. To ID these energy impostors, heed this advice from the experts.

Go sour on sugar. Yes, sugar does give you a fast energy fix—but you end up paying for it. As the sugar floods your bloodstream, your pancreas responds by pumping out more insulin, which sweeps the sugar out of your bloodstream and into cells. As a result, your blood sugar level dips, so you feel pooped and may even get an overwhelming urge for a nap.

Nutritionists recommend limiting daily sugar intake to just 10 percent of calories. That means that if you eat 2,000 calories a day, only 200 of those calories should come from sugar. That's about the amount in a small slice of apple pie.

Forgo fat. Trying to get a kick-start from a fatty meal is like trying to start a campfire with a wet newspaper. Your body has to work hard to digest fatty foods. The process actually slows blood circulation, which impairs the delivery of oxygen to cells. That's when fatigue sets in.

Maximum-Energy Menu

To keep going strong all day long, you need a high-octane meal plan—like this one, designed by Elizabeth Somer, R.D., author of *Nutrition for Women* and *Food and Mood*. It fulfills all the requirements of eating for energy, combining protein- and carbohydrate-rich foods in six small meals spread throughout the day. This meal plan also delivers a healthy dose of fatigue-fighting iron while trimming stamina-sapping sugar, fat, and caffeine.

Breakfast: Toasted bagel topped with 1 tablespoon of peanut butter; banana; 8 ounces of skim milk

Midmorning snack: Bran muffin topped with 2 tablespoons of apple butter; 8 ounces of skim milk

Lunch: 3 ounces of extra-lean roast beef on a whole-wheat roll with tomato, lettuce, and mustard; 1 cup of raw cauliflower florets, sliced carrots, and broccoli; piece of fruit

Midafternoon snack: 6 ounces of vanilla low-fat yogurt sprinkled with ⅓ cup of low-fat granola and 2 tablespoons of dried cranberries, raisins, chopped dates, or other dried fruit

Dinner: 4 to 6 ounces of broiled salmon with dill and lemon; baked potato topped with fat-free sour cream; 1 cup of steamed broccoli; 1 cup of tossed salad with 2 tablespoons of low-fat dressing; ½ cup of fresh blueberries or one-quarter of a honeydew melon

Evening snack: Frozen whole-wheat waffle topped with half of a banana and 1 tablespoon of maple syrup

For a variety of health reasons, many experts recommend that you limit your daily fat intake to 25 percent of calories.

Give joe the cold shoulder. A cup of coffee can get you started in the morning. But drink too much—or too late in the day—and you may find that your get-up-and-go has gotten up and gone. Not only does the caffeine in coffee disrupt your sleep, it also depletes B vitamins and disrupts the absorption of iron—nutrients your body needs to produce energy.

Limit your caffeine consumption to 300 milligrams a day, which is the amount in two 8-ounce cups of coffee, recommends Somer. Or slowly switch to a decaf brew, says Wahida Karmally, R.D, director of nutrition at the Irving Center for Clinical Research at Columbia University in New York City.

Rethink your drink. Don't let those frolicking, fun-loving folks in the beer ads fool you. Alcohol is a sedative, and even though it may give you a little buzz at first, it ultimately drops you like a lead balloon.

Many experts believe that you're better off, health-wise, if you don't drink at all. But if you do drink, keep it moderate—two or three alcoholic beverages a week, at most.

Maximum Mental Performance

Eating to Boost Your Brainpower

As we age, it gets harder and harder to learn new tricks. Our ability to pick up and remember new information starts slowing down as early as our twenties and continues to gradually decline over our lifetimes. "The slowing in memory is tied to the biological deterioration of the nervous system," says Michael Pressley, Ph.D., professor of educational psychology and statistics at the State University of New York at Albany. "You function more slowly as you get older."

Brain Food

But your choice of foods and the nutrients they provide can make you feel years younger, intellectually speaking. Here are some foods researchers think just might help keep our brains in fine form well into old age.

Sprinkle on lecithin. Our brains make a neurotransmitter called acetylcholine (it helps us remember stuff) from the enzyme choline, which is naturally available in the body. Problem is, doctors think our bodies may make less choline as we age. Lecithin is one of the few things we can eat that can help the body secrete more choline.

In one study, 41 people ages 50 to 80 who ate 2 tablespoons (13.5 grams) of lecithin a day forgot fewer names and misplaced fewer things. The top lecithin food sources are liver, egg yolks, and peanuts. Unfortunately, all of those foods also are high in fat and cholesterol, and they're the first foods that people cut out as they become more health-conscious. But lecithin also is plentiful in soybean products.

You also can buy lecithin in granulated form and sprinkle it on cereal, suggests Steven Zeisel, M.D., Ph.D., chairman of the nutrition department at the University of North Carolina at Chapel Hill.

Eat more boron. Boron, found in fruits, nuts, and vegetables, is not considered an essential nutrient, but researchers have found that it may help boost brainpower. One study found that people who ate 3.25 milligrams of the micronutrient a day—roughly ¾ cup of peanuts—scored better on manual dexterity, eye-hand coordination, attention, memory, and perception tests than those who didn't.

Think before you drink. It's true: Alcohol kills brain cells. Researchers studying corpses have found that brains of alcohol abusers weigh less than brains of nonalcoholics. Years of excessive drinking leaves brains with less white matter and cerebral cells. Only a couple of drinks a day over a period of years can reduce your intelligence and memory.

Eat breakfast. Brains need fuel to think. You might be able to skip breakfast and cruise through the morning, but you're in for a huge crash in the afternoon, says Elizabeth Somer, R.D., author of *Nutrition for Women* and *Food and Mood*.

Snack in the afternoon. Here's one you should like. A study conducted at Tufts University in Medford, Massachusetts, found that eating in midafternoon—whether it's yogurt or a chocolate candy bar—increased students' memory and attention skills. Before you reach for that candy bar, though, you should know that students who ate the yogurt did even better than those who had the sugar snack.

Do a slow burn on sugar. It's true. Sugar gives you a quick boost, but it also dumps directly into your bloodstream. The sudden increase in blood sugar causes your body to produce insulin, which makes your blood sugar drop. The result: You get tired.

Instead of candy bars, eat fruit. It contains fructose, but that's a different kind of sugar. The body has to first break down fructose before it can burn it for energy. The sugar is released into the blood slowly, more evenly, and over a longer time, says James M. Rippe, M.D., associate professor of medicine and director of the Center for Clinical and Lifestyle Research at Tufts University Medical School in Shrewsbury, Massachusetts.

Take a coffee break. Caffeine can be a mind-accelerating mood booster when taken in moderation at the right time, says Judith Wurtman, Ph.D., nutrition research scientist at the Massachusetts Institute of Technology in Cambridge, in her book, *Managing Your Mind and Mood through Food*. "There is this tremendous genetic variability among people about how sensitive they are to caffeine," Dr. Rippe says. "They have to find out what amount of coffee fits with who they are genetically."

Hold your intake to no more than two 5-ounce cups of java a day. If you drink more, it's likely the coffee will actually make you more tired than alert in the long run, Somer says. And space it out. Your body is most sensitive to caffeine after it hasn't had it in a while, says Dr. Wurtman. To start your day in top mental form, she recommends drinking a cup of caffeinated coffee soon after getting up in the morning. A cup in midafternoon will also reawaken your brain and help power your mind for another 6 hours or so.

Look to the sea. You might have heard that fish is brain food. And that's somewhat true. Some fish have nutrients that are good for your brain. Tuna has important B vitamins, which can help improve your cognitive skills and memory. And oysters and herring are packed with zinc, which also can help prevent memory loss.

Beating Stress

Staying in the Kitchen When the Heat's On

Stress takes a toll on our bodies. It reduces our absorption and increases our excretion of nutrients. Because we're losing nutrients, we especially need to eat well when stressed out. Unfortunately, it's when we eat our worst.

Instead of eating cereal for breakfast, we grab doughnuts on the way to work. Instead of eating a healthful lunch, we get French fries and a burger on the run at a fast-food joint. Or we skip meals altogether.

"The biggest problem people get into when they are busy is that they violate normal nutrition," says James M. Rippe, M.D., associate professor of medicine and director of the Center for Clinical and Lifestyle Research at Tufts University Medical School in Shrewsbury, Massachusetts.

Stress-Blasting Strategies

Here are some ways to help you conquer stress.

Arm yourself. "Go into an expected stressful situation well-armed," says Elizabeth Somer, R.D., author of *Nutrition for Women* and *Food and Mood*. "What you want to do is boost up your nutrient stores. Have a well-stocked antioxidant system and strong immune system based on a good intake of all the vitamins and minerals. Then when stress hits you from the backside, you're going into it fully armed."

Plan ahead. Bring healthy snacks along. That way, when you get the stress munchies, you won't have to rely on vending machines or fast food. "Bring some healthy food, like apples, rather than candy bars," suggests Dr. Rippe.

Get some help. When Dr. Rippe asked busy executives how they manage to eat nutritionally during times of stress, the most successful ones had someone by their side. If you can get someone (hint: spouse) to pack some turkey sandwiches and carrot sticks for you on the really busy days, you'll have an easier time eating well. Just make sure you return the favor.

Carbo-load to calm down. Sometimes when

Sleeping Through Stress

Can't sleep because of that presentation you have to make in the morning? A low-fat, low-calorie carbohydrate snack should help put you out, says Judith Wurtman, Ph.D., nutrition research scientist at the Massachusetts Institute of Technology in Cambridge and author of *Managing Your Mind and Mood through Food*. According to Dr. Wurtman, here are some snacks that should work as sleeping pills.

- 1½ cups of breakfast cereal without milk
- 1½ ounces of caramel-coated popcorn
- Three fig bars
- Six ginger snaps
- One cinnamon raisin English muffin
- One ⅝-ounce package of cinnamon spice instant oatmeal
- One toaster-size frozen waffle with 1 tablespoon of maple syrup

we're stressed out, it's too obvious. We sweat. Our hands shake. Our tongues get parched. When you really just need to calm down, think carbohydrate. Eating carbohydrates makes our brains produce the calming chemical serotonin. So if stress is getting the best of your nerves, find a quiet place and have a low-fat carbohydrate snack. Snacks that involve crunching or sucking are especially soothing. Think popcorn, rice cakes, cereal, lollipops, frozen pops, and sour balls.

You can even precalm yourself. Eat some carbohydrates about a half-hour before a situation you think
will be stressful, advises Judith Wurtman, Ph.D., nutrition research scientist at the Massachusetts Institute of
Technology in Cambridge and author of *Managing
Your Mind and Mood through Food* . You'll need about
1½ ounces of carbohydrates—two cups of Cheerios—
for the calming effect to take place, Dr. Wurtman says.

Water your brain. Even if you don't show it out-
wardly, that doesn't mean you're not sweating. The average office worker loses 10 cups of fluid a day. And
your brain is the first organ affected by dehydration,
says Paul J. Rosch, M.D., clinical professor of medicine
and psychiatry at New York Medical College in Yonkers,
and president of the American Institute of Stress.

Oftentimes, your body needs water well before
your tongue starts telling you to get a drink. So if
you're feeling tired or stressed, it might be because
you're dehydrated, Dr. Rosch says. Caffeinated beverages rob more water from your body than they replace. For every cup of coffee, you should drink two
glasses of water.

Eat more fiber. Stress plays havoc with our digestive systems. Some researchers advise that when you
are under stress, you should eat at least five servings of
fiber-rich fruits and vegetables, six servings of 100 percent whole-grain breads and cereals, and a serving of
cooked dried peas or beans to keep your digestion running smoothly. But Dr. Rosch cautions that even though
eating more fiber and fruit can improve general health,
some people with irritable bowel syndrome may not
benefit from adding more fiber to their diets.

Take a multivitamin. When the pressure's on,
your nutritional requirements may increase. If, despite

your best intentions, you still don't eat right, multivitamin tablets are there as a backup. Look for one that gives you 100 percent of the RDA for all vitamins and minerals, especially the B vitamins, calcium, magnesium, chromium, copper, iron, manganese, molybdenum, selenium, and zinc.

Take a walk. Instead of reaching for a cigarette, candy bar, or soda, take a walk. "For people who are highly anxious, simply taking a walk will give them an immediate and significant reduction in stress," Dr. Rippe says. "Most people feel the benefit they're getting from walking is not just the exercise but also the time out. You're getting away from the stressful environment."

Beauty Secrets

Foods for Better Skin and Hair

Wander into one of those bath-and-beauty boutiques at the mall, and you'll find shampoos made from kiwifruit, creams made from cucumbers, soaps made from almonds, and lotions made from mangoes. You might get the impression that you're standing before an upscale salad bar rather than a cosmetics counter.

Despite the elaborate packaging, these products press into service hair- and skin-care treatments that have been around for centuries. Even today, women in many parts of the world rely on Mother Nature to keep them looking their best. But you don't have to wear your food to reap its beauty benefits. There's compelling evidence that eating the right stuff—nutritious edibles such as cauliflower, fish, berries, and yogurt—can reward you with healthy hair, glowing skin, elegant nails, and more. It can also help protect against common conditions ranging from acne to wrinkles.

So instead of spending a small fortune on a veritable buffet of potions, why not achieve beauty naturally, from the inside out? The following food strategies can keep you in the pink, from the hair on your head to the nails on your toes.

Acne: Zits Aren't for Kids

You never thought you'd have to deal with one again. Yet here you are, poking and prodding the flaming red pimple that has sprouted on your chin. Sure, you wouldn't mind reliving your youth, but this is a bit too much.

As many adults know all too well, acne doesn't automatically disappear with your teenage years. In fact, some people experience their first breakouts as adults. Others develop rosacea, a condition characterized by pustules and enlarged blood vessels on the nose, cheeks, and forehead.

For blemish-free skin, heed this advice from the experts.

Sail away from seafood. Foods rich in iodine, including clams, crabs, and other shellfish, can cause some people to break out. So if you're acne-prone, leave these off your plate.

Cut out other culprits, too. Scientists have yet to prove that candy, chocolate, or greasy food causes acne. Yet many people swear that they get pimples when they eat too much of this stuff. If that's the case, experts say, then by all means avoid the offending edibles. "These aren't the most healthy foods anyway, so you're better off without them," says D'Anne Kleinsmith, M.D., a dermatologist affiliated with William Beaumont Hospital in West Bloomfield, Michigan.

Zap zits with zinc. The mineral zinc appears to deflate breakouts, perhaps because of its anti-inflammatory properties. Not everyone in the medical community is convinced that zinc works, but it can't hurt to get a little extra in your diet. Good food sources include wheat germ and nonfat or low-fat yogurt.

Age Spots: Calling Cards from Old Sol

These freckle-like brown splotches are your skin's attempt to protect itself from overexposure to the sun by producing too much melanin, or skin pigment. They're usually harmless, although you should see your doctor if you notice any change in their size, color, or texture.

To keep your skin spotless, give the following tips a try.

Lean toward E. "Vitamin E is an anti-inflammatory, and it reduces sun damage to your skin," says Karen E. Burke, M.D., Ph.D., dermatologic surgeon and dermatologist in private practice in New York City. To get more of the vitamin in your diet, choose foods such as wheat germ, mangoes, and safflower, corn, and soybean oils.

Seek out selenium. "Selenium can also minimize sun damage to your skin," Dr. Burke says. Excellent food sources include tuna and baked tortilla chips.

Limit limes. Certain fruits and vegetables—especially limes, celery, parsnips, and carrots—contain psoralens, chemicals that can increase your sensitivity to the sun. Not everyone experiences a reaction after eating these foods. But if you do, even handling them can make you more susceptible to burning. That's why experts recommend washing your hands before venturing out. And be careful about drinking lime-garnished beverages when you're out in the sun.

Cold Sores: Beat Them to the Punch

Call them cold sores or fever blisters. Either way, they hurt like the dickens—and they don't look very nice, either.

Cold sores don't automatically follow a cold: You must first be exposed to a virus called herpes simplex type 1. (Type 2 causes genital herpes.) Once you have the virus, it stays with you for life. Most of the time, it keeps a low profile. But an aggravating factor—perhaps stress, illness, the onset of menstruation, or even a dental procedure—can trigger an outbreak.

The sores themselves usually occur around the mouth, although they've been known to show up inside the nose, on the fingers, and even on the eyelids. They start out as blisters, then break down into scabby lesions. It can take a week to 10 days for an entire episode to run its course.

Fortunately, cold sores tend to announce their impending arrival with a tingling sensation at the site of the eruption. That's your cue to take action. Here's what you can do.

Load up on lysine. An amino acid, lysine suppresses the growth of the herpes simplex virus, thus reducing the number of outbreaks. You can increase your lysine intake by consuming plenty of nonfat and low-fat dairy products, and fruits such as apples and pears.

Avoid arginine. The herpes simplex virus needs arginine, another amino acid, in order to replicate. In some people, very small amounts of arginine can trigger outbreaks. So if you're prone to cold sores, try cutting back on the arginine-rich foods in your diet, including foods made from sesame seeds, peanuts, and soybeans. Then see if you notice any difference in the frequency or severity of your outbreaks.

Fingernail Problems: A Sign That Something Is Amiss

Have you taken a good, hard look at your fingernails lately? If not, perhaps you should. You see, your nails are built-in barometers of your body's nutrition status. When they become brittle or misshapen, it usually means that you're getting too little—or too much—of a particular nutrient.

Experts recommend the following strategies for healthy, sharp-looking nails.

Get a boost from biotin. A member of the B-vitamin family, biotin helps to build strong nails. In fact, researchers in Switzerland found that 2,500 micrograms of biotin a day could increase nail thickness by 25 percent.

The dose of biotin used in the Swiss study is more than eight times the Daily Value (DV), which is 300 micrograms. You can boost your intake of the vitamin by consuming soybean flour, cauliflower, lentils, and skim or low-fat (1 percent) milk.

Iron out the problem. If your nails appear spoon-shaped, you may have iron-deficiency anemia. You should see your doctor for a proper diagnosis. But in the meantime, try to get more iron-rich foods in your diet. Good sources include lean meat, Cream of Wheat cereal, baked potatoes, soybeans, and tofu.

Shed pounds slowly. Crash dieting can take a toll on your fingernails, leaving them riddled with horizontal ridges. If you want to lose weight, experts advise, don't eat so little that you lose more than 2 pounds a week.

Skin Cancer: Fry Now, Pay Later

Despite all the warnings about the sun's damaging ultraviolet rays, many people still cling to the notion that a bronzed body is the epitome of health and beauty. They don't seem to realize that every minute spent in pursuit of the perfect tan increases their risk of skin cancer. This form of cancer is the most common in the United States, accounting for 40 percent of all diagnosed cancer cases.

Obviously, the best thing you can do for your skin's sake is to limit the amount of time you spend in the sun. When you do venture out, be sure to wear a sunscreen with a sun protection factor (SPF) of 15 or higher. Beyond that, you can try the following dietary strategies for a little extra insurance against skin cancer.

Get your fill of fish. There's some evidence that omega-3 fatty acids, found in fish such as mackerel and salmon, can help prevent skin cancer. Researchers at Baylor College of Medicine in Houston found that people who consume large amounts of omega-3's every day have less chance of developing the kind of cell damage associated with skin cancer during exposure to ultraviolet light, compared with people who don't consume large amounts of omega-3's.

Take time for tea. Laboratory research suggests that drinking green tea can reduce skin cancer risk. Scientists suspect that the tea's anticancer effects come from compounds called polyphenols. Like beta-carotene and vitamins C and E, polyphenols are antioxidants, which means that they protect cells from damage caused by radiation and other toxins. You can buy green tea in supermarkets and health food stores.

Eat lean. When a group of volunteers with histories of skin cancer followed a low-fat diet, they had fewer cancerous growths over a 2-year period than a similar group that consumed twice as much fat. Scientists suspect that certain components in fat may cause skin cells to mutate in harmful ways. For this and other health reasons, many experts recommend limiting your daily fat intake to no more than 25 percent of calories.

Thinning Hair: Not for Men Only

Eating right might not be a cure for the type of balding men undergo, but it can help women. At least 25 percent of women have a problem with thinning hair, Dr. Kleinsmith says. Usually it's only temporary—the possible result of crash dieting, stress, or hormonal changes. Under these conditions, the right diet can help a woman keep her tresses in tip-top shape. Here's what the experts recommend.

Eye your iron intake. Iron-deficiency anemia can result in hair loss. To make sure that you're meeting the DV of 18 milligrams, pile your plate with iron-rich foods, suggests Mary Frances Picciano, Ph.D., professor of nutrition at Pennsylvania State University in University Park. Lean meat is perhaps the best source of the mineral. Other choices include Cream of Wheat cereal, baked potatoes, soybeans, and tofu.

Sup sensibly. Radical weight-loss programs can deprive your body of the nutrients it needs to function properly, and that can lead to thinning hair. If you want to lose weight, do it slowly and steadily—no more than 2 pounds a week. And hold your daily fat consumption to no more than 25 percent of calories.

Varicose Veins: Not Inevitable

Imagine pushing a car uphill with its brakes on and you get a pretty good idea of what your blood is up against as it makes the journey from your legs to your heart. Valves, the gatelike structures in your veins, keep blood moving in the right direction. But sometimes a valve fails to shut properly—the result of too much sitting or standing. When that happens, blood pools in your leg, causing the vein to bulge toward the surface of your skin. That's what you know as a varicose vein.

What you eat—and what you don't eat—can influence whether you develop varicose veins. You can reduce your risk by heeding this advice from the experts.

Fight back with fiber. When you strain hard to move your bowels, you create pressure in your abdomen. That causes blood to back up into your legs, and this, over time, weakens vein walls.

To prevent constipation, include plenty of fiber-rich foods in your meals. Some top-notch sources are beans, whole grains, fruits, and vegetables. Some particularly high-fiber foods to look for include chickpeas and dried pears.

Pick some berries. Deep-colored berries such as cherries, blueberries, and blackberries contain chemical compounds called bioflavonoids. Scientists believe that bioflavonoids make tiny capillaries less likely to distend or break down, preventing the appearance of so-called spider veins on the surface of the skin. Other good sources of bioflavonoids include grape juice and the white membranes of citrus fruits.

Go easy with the saltshaker. A too-high salt intake can cause your legs to swell. And that puts a lot of pressure on your veins if they are already damaged.

Wrinkles: Foods That Fight Father Time

Were it not for the sun, our skin would stay relatively wrinkle-free until we reach our seventies. Instead, most of us start noticing smile lines and crow's-feet years earlier, thanks to photoaging. In fact, at least 80 percent of the skin changes we see as we get older are the result of excessive sun exposure.

By adulthood, some damage has already been done. But don't sit around and wait for wrinkles to appear—there's plenty you can do to delay them. For starters, limit the time you spend in the sun—and when you are outside, protect your skin with sunscreen of at least SPF 15. Then round out your wrinkle-reducing plan with these nutrition strategies.

Up the ante. At least one study of animals has shown that exposure to ultraviolet rays depletes levels of vitamins C and E. These nutrients are antioxidants; they protect your cells from the damage caused by radiation and other toxins. Fortunately, you can easily restock your body's antioxidant supply: For vitamin C, choose oranges, broccoli, kiwifruit, and peppers. Wheat germ and vegetable oils (safflower, corn, and soybean) have generous supplies of vitamin E.

Stay afloat. Remember to drink lots of water. Most experts recommend at least eight 8-ounce glasses a day. If you perspire a lot, you should aim even higher.

No More Diet Daze

An Eating Strategy That Works

We live in a country that honors hot dogs and apple pie as its national cuisine. Is it any wonder, then, that dieting now rivals baseball as America's favorite pastime?

At this very moment, one out of three people in America is waging a battle of the bulge. In fact, the average woman tries at least 10 diets in her lifetime—cutting calories, popping pills, slurping shakes, and even forgoing food completely. Often the pounds do disappear. But, for most people, some or all eventually creep back.

Yet plenty of Americans manage to achieve and maintain a healthy weight. How do they do it? Simple: They stop dieting. Many experts agree that you should do the same. "We don't use the word *diet*," says Maria Simonson, Sc.D., Ph.D., professor emeritus and director of the health, weight, and stress clinic at the Johns Hopkins Medical Institutions in Baltimore. "It sends a shiver down people's spines. We say *eating program*."

Why the trade-off in terminology? Because most of us associate "diet" with giving up favorite foods and going hungry. That's why dieting doesn't work.

Never Say Diet

If you are carrying some extra pounds, you have a very good reason for wanting to send them packing.

You see, being overweight puts you at risk for some serious health problems. Research shows that even a relatively modest weight gain—say, 20 pounds—can double your risk of a heart attack. Other studies have linked overweight to gallstones, gout, high blood pressure, high cholesterol, diabetes, stroke, and cancers of the endometrium (uterine lining) and in women, possibly the breast.

So unloading the excess baggage is a good thing. It's the way we usually go about it that sets us up for failure. Many of us skip meals, and when we do eat, we skimp on portions. Sure, you lose weight, but you also end up with a body that craves sustenance.

When you don't feed your body enough, it slips into famine mode and starts hoarding the fat that you're trying so hard to get rid of. You don't burn as many calories as usual, as your metabolism shifts into low gear.

Restrict your food intake often enough, and you also become more susceptible to episodes of binge eating. Scientists theorize that as you train yourself to ignore your internal hunger cues, you more easily respond to external cues, which could be anything from a rough day to a television commercial for your favorite fast food.

In short, you simply can't starve yourself slim. If you try, you're likely to end up carrying more pounds, not less.

Fat and Figures

If eating less food doesn't help you to lose weight, try eating less fat. By sticking with nonfat and low-fat foods, you can actually eat more and still drop those persistent pounds.

To prove this point, researchers at Cornell University in Ithaca, New York, had a group of volunteers alternate between a low-fat and a "regular," full-fat eating plan. Except for fat content, the foods were identical in both plans. The volunteers lost ½ pound per week when they ate low-fat. Just as important, they reported that they didn't even feel as though they were dieting.

As a weight-loss strategy, cutting fat intake works for a couple of reasons. First of all, fat packs a lot of calories: You get 9 calories in a gram of fat, compared with 4 in a gram of carbohydrate or protein. What's more, your body loves to store fat because the process demands so little energy. Just 3 percent of fat calories get burned as they're moved into storage, compared with 23 percent of carbohydrate or protein calories.

How Much Do You Need?

No matter how hard you might try, you couldn't possibly eliminate all the fat from your eating plan. Nor would you want to, says Joanne Curran-Celentano, R.D., Ph.D., associate professor of nutritional sciences at the University of New Hampshire in Durham. Your body needs some fat just to keep itself running. Besides, a certain amount of fat makes food taste good. If you cut back on fat too much, you aren't going to enjoy your food, which means that you'll probably abandon your good intentions at the first opportunity.

The problem is that most of us consume more fat than we need to—a lot more. The average intake in this country stands at about 35 percent of calories. By comparison, many experts consider 25 percent of calories the standard for good health. Some believe that you should aim even lower—say, 20 percent of calories—to lose weight.

Let's suppose that you're consuming 1,800 calories a day. Applying the 20 percent guideline, no more than 360 of those calories should come from fat. Since 1 gram of fat has 9 calories, you should eat no more than 40 grams of fat a day.

Of course, this raises another question: Just how many calories do you need every day? Here's a simple formula: First determine your activity level. (Your activity level is important because exercise burns calories, which means they don't get stored as fat.) Give yourself a 12 if your lifestyle involves light walking at most and you exercise only occasionally; a 15 if your job requires light walking or you get 30 to 60 minutes of aerobic exercise three times a week; or an 18 if you are very active and exercise for at least 60 minutes four or more times a week. Determine your calorie needs by multiplying your activity level score by your weight in pounds. (If you're overweight, multiply your activity level score by your goal weight. A healthy weight-loss goal is ½ to 1 pound per week.)

Livin' Lean

Shifting the focus of your weight-loss efforts to dietary fat can take some getting used to. But don't think for a minute that sacrifice is the price to be paid for becoming slender and shapely. Simply reducing your daily intake of butter, margarine, or oil by 1 tablespoon will leave you 10 pounds lighter in a year—even if you do nothing else to lose weight.

To further trim the fat from your eating habits, try these tips.

Document the details. You can't begin cutting back on fat until you know where it's coming from. That's why many experts recommend keeping a food diary for at least a few days. It doesn't have to be anything fancy—just write down what you've eaten immediately after each meal or snack.

A food diary serves two purposes. First, it helps you to spot the "hidden" fat in the course of a day's worth of eating—like the handful of peanuts you grab in the break room or the glass of whole milk you drink at bedtime. Second, it shows you at a glance which foods you might be most comfortable deleting from your menu, says Ronette Kolotkin, Ph.D., director of behavioral programs at the Duke University Diet and Fitness Center in Durham, North Carolina.

Go slowly. Once you've identified each food that is inflating your fat budget, you have several options: You can look for a nonfat or low-fat version, you can eat less of it, or you can eliminate it from your menu altogether. Whichever option you choose, focus on just one or two foods at a time. If you try to overhaul your eating habits in one fell swoop, you're just setting yourself up for problems.

Remember, too, that it takes at least 13 weeks to become acclimated to low-fat eating. Patience is the key to your success.

Learn label lingo. The label on a packaged food can be your greatest ally in the battle of the bulge—if you know how to interpret all those numbers. They don't necessarily mean what you think.

Take, for example, the percentage of calories from fat. You'd probably assume—quite reasonably—that this figure is based on the number of calories in the food. But it's not. Instead, it's based on 2,000 calories—an entire day's intake. Depending on your size and activity level, you may need less or more.

For more accurate indicators of a food's fat content, check out the number of fat grams and the number of calories from fat per serving.

Roll up the welcome mat. If your goal is to eat less fat, you can do yourself a big favor by banning fat-laden goodies from your kitchen. In fact, now is the ideal time to do a little housecleaning: Go through your refrigerator, cupboards, and pantry, getting rid of all the bad stuff to make room for the good stuff.

Tip the Scale in Your Favor

Bringing your fat intake to a healthy level can work wonders for your waistline. But there's a lot more you can do to peel off those extra pounds and keep them off. The following strategies will help you whip your eating habits into shape and make you a weight-loss winner.

Consider calories. This is absolutely critical. "Many people think that they can eat as much low-fat food as they want, but these foods contain a significant number of calories," says Simone French, Ph.D., assistant professor of epidemiology at the University of Minnesota in Minneapolis. "And if you take in a lot more calories than you need—even if they're fat-free calories—you gain weight."

For every 3,500 "unused" calories that you consume, you gain 1 pound. On the other hand, if you cut your calorie intake by 100 calories a day, you can lose 10 pounds over the course of a year—even if you make no other changes in your eating habits.

Keep those carbs coming. Your body would much rather burn carbohydrate calories than attempt to store them as fat. Indeed, research has shown that people who achieve and maintain a healthy weight consume an abundance of complex carbohydrates, including foods such as pasta, bread, beans, rice, and potatoes.

What makes complex carbohydrates so figure-friendly? For starters, they have low energy densities—that is, they weigh a lot, but they contain relatively few calories, according to Barbara Rolls, Ph.D., professor of nutrition at Pennsylvania State University in University Park. Foods that have low energy densities can fill you up without filling you out, she explains.

Complex carbohydrates also switch off hunger by triggering nerve endings to alert your brain that you're full. With high-fat foods, this message never gets delivered, and you end up eating more than you should.

Of course, not all complex carbohydrates are created equal. Go easy on foods such as packaged baked goods, which are usually made with refined flour and pack a lot of fat and sugar to boot. Stick with whole grains, fruits, and vegetables, Dr. Rolls suggests. "They're virtually fat-free, they contain a lot of nutrients, and they fill you up."

Become a fan of fiber. Foods that are high in fiber create a feeling of fullness, so you tend to eat less of them. "It's a good idea to select high-fiber foods as your carbohydrates," Dr. Curran-Celentano says. "You'll get more nutrients and avoid dips in blood sugar, which can cause food cravings and hunger pangs." Many experts recommend consuming up to 35 grams of fiber a day. Choose whole-grain cereals, beans, fruits, and vegetables.

Drown your hunger. Many experts agree that plain old H_2O is the best appetite suppressant around. When you give your body water, it thinks it has been fed and so stops bugging you for food. In fact, often what you perceive as hunger is really thirst in disguise. To stay well-hydrated and stave off a grumbly stomach, try to drink at least eight 8-ounce glasses of water a day.

Go easy on the alcohol. You get 106 calories in 5 ounces of wine and 150 calories in 12 ounces of beer. If you have more than one of either, you can really pack in the calories—and eventually, you'll pack on the pounds. There's also evidence that alcohol interferes with your body's fat-burning process, which makes it harder to lose weight. Try not to exceed three drinks a week.

Mind your mealtimes. Skipping meals can be hazardous to your waistline. Besides leaving you famished and vulnerable to overeating, it also slows down your metabolism. In fact, research has shown that people who bypass breakfast burn about 5 percent fewer calories than people who eat at least three meals a day.

Divide and conquer. Instead of sticking with the

standard three squares, make the switch to mini-meals—five or six small meals spread over the course of a day. This style of eating has a couple of advantages, weight loss–wise. For one thing, you never get too hungry, since you're feeding your body every few hours. For another, you avoid taking in too many calories in one sitting.

Linger over dinner. When you eat something, your brain doesn't get the message for about 20 minutes, says Susan Olson, Ph.D., clinical psychologist and weight management consultant in Seattle and author of *Keeping It Off: Winning at Weight Loss*. This delay means that you can get full before you actually *feel* full. Taking the time to savor every morsel of your meal can prevent you from overeating.

Know the source. Here's another little trick of the weight-loss trade: Be careful to distinguish between hunger and appetite. Hunger is driven by a genuine physical need for food. Appetite, on the other hand, often grows from your emotions. Weight-loss experts call it head hunger: You eat because you want to, not because you have to.

To help sharpen your hunger awareness, try this exercise at your next meal. Before you start eating, rate your hunger on a scale of 0 to 5 (0 being the least hungry, 5 being the most). Eat one-quarter of the food on your plate, then rate your hunger. Wait 5 minutes, then rate your hunger again. Repeat the sequence. As you concentrate on the process of eating, you just may discover that you're satisfied before you even clean your plate.

Choose foods that satisfy. Researchers at the University of Sydney in Australia put together a list of "bargain foods" that, calorie for calorie, have the greatest potential to satisfy your hunger. The highest-scoring food? The baked potato. It gives you the most bang for your caloric buck, filling you up faster and on fewer calories than any other food tested. Rounding out the top five are fish, oatmeal, oranges, and apples. At the bottom of the satiety barrel: croissants, cake, doughnuts, candy bars, and peanuts.

Hot and Cold Weather

Setting Your Own Climate Control

Researchers at Johns Hopkins University in Baltimore have studied our weather-related eating habits for years. And they have us pretty well figured out. In the summer when our bodies have switched to a low-calorie burning mode, we eat lots of raw vegetables, drink plenty of fluids, and chow on carbohydrates and sweets.

In the winter we switch to fat and protein. We eat a lot more and a lot more often, and we put on weight.

"We find appetites usually increase in winter for psychological and physiological reasons," says Maria Simonson, Sc.D., Ph.D., professor emeritus and director of the health, weight, and stress clinic at Johns Hopkins Medical Institutions in Baltimore. "You're going to eat more even if you're snugly inside, because food has the psychological effect of making us feel more secure and protected from the bad weather outside."

In the Summertime

If you don't pay attention, the weather will control your diet. Here are a few ways to outsmart Mother Nature when the heat is on.

Drink water. You know this. But we're going to tell you again because—if you're like most of us—you don't do it. Even though it's common sense, few of us drink enough water. It's especially important in the summer when you are losing a lot of fluid by sweating. And sweating, after all, is your body's cooling system. Make sure to drink about eight 8-ounce glasses of liquid a day, says Neva Cochran, R.D., a private nutrition consultant and a spokesperson for the American Dietetic Association in Dallas.

Don't scream for ice cream. Drinking really cold drinks or eating something cold such as ice cream might make you feel cooler for about 15 minutes, but they won't cool your body. Body heat is controlled by calories. So when you have a cold, high-calorie snack such as a milk shake or ice cream, you're going to make yourself hotter.

"Ice cream will give you more body heat than the warmth that lasts 10 or 15 minutes from a hot bowl of soup because the calories are higher," Dr. Simonson says.

Avoid dressing up. Many people like to drink a lot of fruit juice and eat cold-cut salads with oily dressings in the summer. It just seems like light eating, but it's not. Oily dressings are packed with fat calories, and many fruit drinks are loaded with sugar calories.

Weathering Winter

There's something to be said for foraging outside in the Arctic region: food. You can eat and eat and eat without gaining weight. That's because it's so cold your body needs about 7,000 calories a day just to keep you warm.

Theoretically, winter is the best time to lose weight. Realistically, however, most of us gain pounds between October and April. Why? For one, we usually stay in the heated indoors during the winter. And even though we do need extra calories, we tend to eat much more than we need. Here are some ways to keep off winter weight gain and stay warm.

Switch to snacking. Instead of eating three big winter meals a day, have five smaller ones. The constant calories will make you feel warmer, and spreading them out will help you control your weight. "If you have a habit of eating more and more frequent meals, less of what you eat will turn to fat," Dr. Simonson says.

Stay active. If you keep up activity in winter, you will be able to keep weight down. "It requires a lot more energy and more effort to generate body heat. Besides, you wear more clothes in winter, and that increases your energy expenditure," Dr. Simonson says.

Cut the fat. You're going to crave fat and protein in the winter. It's okay to go with the protein. It will help you stay warm. But forget the fat. Go for lean meats, poultry, and fish to satisfy your cravings, says Dr. Simonson.

Remove temptation. When you're cooped up in the house, you might linger around the kitchen table.

Fire Up Your Metabolism

To burn calories, why not add a little fire to your food? Seasoning your meals with sizzling spices can actually boost your metabolic rate and melt away the pounds.

In a study at Oxford-Brooks University in England, researchers had people eat two meals—one bland, the other spiked with hot mustard and chili sauce. While both meals boosted metabolism (your body expends energy to digest all types of food), the spicy cuisine sent it soaring 25 percent higher. And it stayed elevated for about 3 hours after the last fiery bite.

Chili powder, chili peppers, horseradish, and hot-pepper sauce can rev up your metabolic engine, too. You can tell that they're working when you start to perspire.

While you're at it, you might want to dampen those flames with some ice-cold water. Your body has to expend energy to heat the H_2O to 98.6°F, your normal temperature. Drinking eight 8-ounce glasses a day burns 123 calories. And all you have to do is swallow.

Instead of letting snack foods stare you in the face, keep them locked up in a dark cupboard. Or don't buy them until the spring thaw. Instead, make sure more nutritious, lower-fat items such as grapes and oranges are within reach, suggests Dr. Simonson.

Drink up. Instead of eating every time you feel

the urge to snack, have something to drink. Liquids move to your intestines faster than solid food and they make you feel fuller sooner. Liquid intake is important in the winter because your body can easily become dehydrated as it works extra hard to moisten and warm the cold air you inhale, says Cochran.

Pretend it's summer. You're better off sticking to lighter, summer-style eating during the winter. Have soup and salad nights. Make it a hearty soup like chicken or vegetable or bean. They take longer to eat, says Dr. Simonson, so your brain has a chance to register that your stomach is full before you overeat.

PART 4

Home Alone with the Refrigerator

Your Food, Your Mood

When Emotions, Not Hunger, Make You Eat

For most of us, it all began sometime in childhood. We'd fall and scrape a knee, and our moms would console us with a big bowl of ice cream. Or we wouldn't get invited to a classmate's birthday party, so Grandma would bake us her special apple pie to cheer us up.

Experiences like these taught us an indelible lesson: Eating makes us feel good. We learned early on to use food as salve for our emotional wounds.

So even though we're all grown up now, we still turn to food to soothe bad feelings. It's not that our stomachs are growling. We're attempting to fulfill a different kind of hunger—what Sandra Campbell, Psy.D., clinical director of the eating disorders program at the Brattleboro Retreat in Vermont, calls a hunger of the soul.

We may eat because we're angry, depressed, anxious, or sad. Or because we have low self-esteem. Or even because we're trying to avoid intimacy.

When we allow our emotions to dictate our food choices, our internal hunger cues—the ones driven by a genuine physical need for sustenance—get thrown

How Happy Is Your Diet?

Many of us use food to make us feel good. Unfortunately, we don't always realize that we're doing it. There's double danger in "dining blind." It leads to weight gain because we're overriding our internal hunger cues, but it does nothing to resolve the underlying problem.

The following quiz, developed at the Duke University Medical Center in Durham, North Carolina, can help you determine whether you're an emotional eater. Simply read each question and answer true or false, then tally up your score as noted at the end.

T   F   If someone hurts me or makes me angry, I feel better if I eat something.

T   F   When I feel that my family or friends are disappointed in me, I turn to food for comfort.

T   F   When I have a lot of work pressure, I find myself eating.

T   F   I often find myself eating because I don't have anything else to do.

T   F   I eat fattening food only when I'm alone and others can't see me.

T   F   I overeat when I'm feeling lonely.

T   F   I overeat after an argument with my mate or my boss.

T   F   Sometimes I don't stop eating even though I feel nauseous or I can't breathe.

off track. The brain chemicals that switch hunger on and off become confused. We end up eating more than we should, which ultimately sinks us into an even deeper funk. "It becomes a vicious circle," says Eliza-

T F   I feel very guilty and ashamed when I overeat.

T F   I become panicky if food is not available when I want it.

T F   I'm always thinking about food.

T F   Once I start eating, I can't stop until I finish whatever is in front of me.

T F   My eating is always extreme—I'm either perfectly in control or completely out of control.

What Your Score Means

To determine your score, count up the number of items that you answered "true." Then find the appropriate category below.

0 to 2: For the most part, your eating patterns are unrelated to your emotional state.

3 to 6: You have some emotional-eating tendencies that need to be addressed. Begin to pay attention to the relationship between your emotional needs and your eating patterns.

7 to 13: Food plays a central role in your emotional life. There is a strong relationship between how you feel and how much or what kinds of food you eat. You must learn to better recognize your feelings, separate feelings from food, and find other coping mechanisms besides eating.

beth Somer, R.D., author of *Nutrition for Women* and *Food and Mood*.

Tuning in to our internal hunger cues can help us head off emotion-driven bingeing. Even better, it can help us choose foods that moderate our moods in a positive, healthful way.

It's All in Your Head

You already know that your body breaks down foods and then retains nutrients to fuel its various systems. In much the same way, your brain uses certain substances from foods to produce chemicals that regulate mental functions, including mood, alertness, and memory.

Scientists have identified at least 40 of these chemicals, called neurotransmitters. They fire back and forth between the nerve cells in your brain, enabling the cells to communicate with one another. Having too little or too much of a particular neurotransmitter can alter these signals, paving the way for changes in the way you feel, think, and act. Neurotransmitter deficits and overloads are linked to serious conditions such as depression, mania, and memory loss.

Three of these brain chemicals—serotonin, dopamine, and norepinephrine—influence mood and appetite. "What you eat can dramatically affect the levels of these neurotransmitters—and, therefore, how you feel," Somer says.

Serotonin: Nature's Mood Medicine

Of the three neurotransmitters Somer mentions, serotonin appears to have the strongest effects on mood. "Without enough of it, you can experience symptoms such as food cravings, depression, and insomnia," Somer notes. "How much serotonin you have is often directly related to your diet."

Your brain manufactures serotonin from an

amino acid called tryptophan, found in protein-rich foods such as chicken, tuna, and tofu. Ironically, though, eating these foods actually lowers the level of tryptophan—and serotonin—in your brain, Somer says.

Why? Because protein foods have more than two dozen different amino acids, and every one of them makes a beeline for your brain. Tryptophan is the pokiest of the bunch. Invariably, it ends up getting stuck in your bloodstream.

For tryptophan to complete the journey to your brain, you have to get the other amino acids out of the way. You can do that simply by eating a carbohydrate-rich meal. The carbohydrates trigger the release of the hormone insulin, which escorts the other amino acids into your body's cells. Tryptophan then has the all-clear.

Once it reaches its destination, tryptophan completes its mission by serving as the catalyst to increase serotonin levels. Serotonin has a calming, even tranquilizing effect on your mood. If you're stressed, for instance, serotonin makes you feel relaxed. And if you're already relaxed, serotonin sends you off to Dreamland.

Dopamine and Norepinephrine: Primed for Action

The other two players in the brain game, dopamine and norepinephrine, have an impact on your mental sharpness. They influence your alertness, your thinking skills, and your memory. Still, if levels of these neurotransmitters run low, you may feel depressed or experience other changes in your mood. And if they're too high, they can actually stimulate stress.

To manufacture dopamine and norepinephrine, your brain needs an amino acid called tyrosine—which, coincidentally, is also found in protein-rich foods. Compared to tryptophan, which travels more slowly, tyrosine is a speed demon. It routinely beats out other amino acids in the race for your brain, Somer explains.

Of course, this means that when tyrosine is present, tryptophan—being the slowpoke that it is—doesn't stand a chance in the race. You'll have lots of dopamine and norepinephrine but not so much serotonin. As a result, you'll feel more energized than relaxed.

Are You Really Hungry?

You can see how food choices might cause changes in mood over the course of the day. But this still doesn't explain what drives us to binge on particular foods when we're blue. Why do tough times make us want to bury our noses in the fridge instead of a good book?

Sometimes the urge to eat comes from within. As mentioned earlier, cravings for certain foods may be your body's way of saying that it needs something.

Typically, neurotransmitters—the same ones that govern your mood—work with hormones and your stomach to monitor your body's nutrient status. They're like your own personal pit crew, whose job is to ensure that your body is properly fueled at all times. When something runs low, they'll pull you in for a pit stop. You'll recognize their signal as that familiar grumbling and gnawing in the pit of your stomach. This is what the experts consider true hunger—an honest-to-goodness, biological need for food. It's a basic tool for survival, as instinctive and natural as breathing.

Then there's another type of hunger—what some

weight-loss experts call head hunger. You eat because you want to, not because you have to. Your emotions can fuel head hunger. You may turn to food to elicit good feelings or to wipe out bad feelings. You may even notice a pattern to your head hunger. Over a period of months or even years, you may repeatedly eat the same food in response to a specific negative emotion or circumstance, says Susan Olson, Ph.D., clinical psychologist and weight management consultant in Seattle and author of *Keeping It Off: Winning at Weight Loss*.

Emotions à la Mode

Mastering emotional eating, then, starts with recognizing the difference between physical hunger and head hunger. This takes a little practice, but it's worth the effort. You can stop yourself from bingeing—and learn constructive ways to deal with the problems that are causing your emotional distress.

Understanding how food influences your mood is important, too. When you find yourself facing tough times, you can plan your meals to include foods that leave you feeling calm and relaxed.

The following strategies can help you identify emotion-driven eating patterns and establish more mood-friendly eating habits.

Document your diet. Start to carry a small notebook or a 3- by 5-inch index card in your pocket or purse. Then each time you eat something when you are not physically hungry, make a note of what it is and how you're feeling. Include information about where you are and who, if anyone, is with you.

"We call this monitoring," says Katherine Halmi, M.D., professor of psychiatry at Cornell University

(continued on page 222)

Find Your Food Personality

How would you describe your food personality? Yes, you do have one. Every one of us does. It's shaped by your eating routine, your favorite foods, your beliefs about what constitutes good nutrition, and a host of other factors.

In her work with clients, Susan Olson, Ph.D., clinical psychologist and weight management consultant in Seattle and author of *Keeping It Off: Winning at Weight Loss*, has identified seven basic food personalities. Each is profiled below, along with Dr. Olson's advice for countering it.

Feeler. "When I feel happy, depressed, bored, or angry, turning to food makes me feel very comfortable."

Your strategy: Focus on expressing your feelings in more healthful ways, such as hitting a pillow, listening to music, or calling a friend. Also, try to control your environment. Keep high-fat foods out of your home, for instance.

Human doer. "I eat on the go, and frequently I eat without thinking. I usually have difficulty following a strict eating routine."

Your strategy: Grazing is okay, as long as it's healthy. Learn the nutritious choices and stop feeling guilty if you don't eat the way others do. Also, keep simple finger foods—such as bagels, cut-up carrots, and fruit—on hand.

Thinker. "I'm highly critical of myself, and I can be compulsive in my behavior. If I believe I've made an eating mistake, it will often turn into an all-out binge."

Your strategy: Your goal is to be gentler on yourself and to keep your life balanced. Plan fun things so you don't get too obsessive about eating. Take 10 to 20 minutes a day to listen to a meditation tape, or buy a coloring book and color outside the lines.

Food hedonist. "For me, food is very sensual. I love the look, the smell, and especially the taste of food."

Your strategy: Rechannel your passion for food into other areas, such as reading, crafts, music—even a relationship. If you love to cook, create your own low-fat recipes.

Dreamer. "I want to reach my ideal weight but I'm easily discouraged, and I tend to fall back into counterproductive eating habits."

Your strategy: Work on improving your self-image by focusing on your uniqueness, your positive attributes, and whatever makes you feel good.

"People" person. "I love nothing better than going to a party or having lunch with a friend in a nice restaurant. But I'm always afraid I'll lose control of sensible eating in social situations."

Your strategy: Focus on the human connection and make food secondary. Brush up on the basics of good nutrition so you can make healthful choices in restaurants and other social situations.

Fitness fan. "My body and my health are very important to me—I'll do anything to learn how to feel and look better. But sometimes I can be too compulsive about eating and/or exercising."

Your strategy: You have a definite advantage. You exercise to burn calories and to relieve tension, and you wouldn't deliberately eat something that would harm your health. The trick is to not become so overly obsessive that you ignore other parts of your life.

Medical College in New York City and director of the eating disorder program at New York Hospital, West-chester Division, in White Plains. "You write it all down and look for a pattern."

After a week or so, you may notice that you consistently eat when you're depressed, anxious, angry, bored, or lonely. Or you may use food as a substitute for sex and intimacy.

Consider the reason. Once you've identified an emotional-eating pattern, you can dig a little deeper to disclose the "automatic thoughts" that prompt you to reach for food for comfort or a quick escape.

Suppose, for instance, that you're hosting a party on Saturday night. You worry that you won't have enough food, that no one will talk to each other, that no one will come. Thoughts like these can make you feel anxious or stressed—and they can drive you to binge.

Stick with a schedule. You can also uncover emotional eating patterns by planning your meals and snacks for regular times, say experts. If you eat on a schedule, then find yourself wanting food an hour after lunch, you can say, "Wait. This isn't necessary. What's going on here?"

Choose high-carbohydrate cuisine. During emotionally trying times, your brain quickly uses up its supply of mood-boosting serotonin. And when serotonin is in short supply, negative feelings tend to increase.

Eating foods that are high in complex carbohydrates, including pasta, bagels, and baked potatoes, can raise a low serotonin level, so you feel less stressed and more relaxed. You get a bonus, too: As serotonin increases, appetite usually decreases, which means that you're less likely to eat your way through tough times.

Steer clear of sweets. Eating chocolate, cookies, and other sugary treats can make you feel better pretty quickly, but the effects won't last. In some people, these foods cause blood sugar levels to shoot way up. In response, your pancreas dumps insulin into your bloodstream, which in turn ushers the sugar out of your bloodstream and into cells. Your blood sugar level quickly plummets. This sudden drop can leave you feeling tired and irritable, and it may even trigger a craving, Somer explains.

Trim the fat. Most of us yearn for sweet and fatty or salty and fatty foods. Unfortunately, eating fatty foods seems to prompt cravings for even more fatty foods, according to Sarah Leibowitz, Ph.D., behavioral neurobiologist at Rockefeller University in New York City.

In animal studies, Dr. Leibowitz found that a high-fat diet prompted the production of a neurochemical that stimulates an appetite for fat. For a variety of health-related reasons, many experts advise limiting your daily fat intake to no more than 25 percent of calories.

The Blues Foods

The Do's and Don'ts of Emotional Eating

In the movie *Sleepless in Seattle*, actor Meg Ryan eats her way from one scene to the next. She realizes that she's engaged to the wrong man and devours a bag of potato chips. She falls head over heels for inaccessible Tom Hanks and downs a pint of ice cream. She wallows in her sorrow by watching the classic tearjerker *An Affair to Remember* while shoveling fistfuls of popcorn into her mouth.

Of course, there's a big difference between the "reel" world and the real world. When we routinely eat like that, we can pack on pounds. And we deprive our bodies of vital nutrients because we're replacing healthful foods with "comfort foods" like chocolate, cookies, and ice cream.

Now there's nothing wrong with an occasional indulgence to brighten a blue mood. The key word here is *occasional*. When we habitually use food as emotional anesthesia—when we depend on Ben & Jerry, or Sara Lee, or Mrs. Smith to ease our inner turmoil—we're headed for trouble, says Linda Smolak, Ph.D., professor of psychology at Kenyon College in Gambier, Ohio. Although emotional eating can temporarily numb our woes, in the long run it makes us not only less healthy but less happy, too.

The Need to Feed

Men and women naturally turn to food to ease emotional distress or fill an emotional void. Even men do it, although men seldom feel as guilty about it as women, who tend to be much more conscious of what they consume and how it affects appearance.

But why do people do it? Well, sometimes the need to feed is biologically driven. Scientists believe there's a reason we crave sweets when we're stressed: They are rich in carbohydrates, which supply the raw materials the brain uses to produce serotonin.

Serotonin is the "feel-good" brain chemical that boosts your sense of well-being, explains Dianne Lindewall, Ph.D., supervising behavioral psychologist for the George Washington University Obesity Management Program in Washington, D.C. Because stress rapidly drains your serotonin supply, a craving may be your body's way of recouping its losses.

Often, though, emotional eating is a response to external rather than internal cues. In other words, rather than eating because our bodies tell us to, we eat because we're anxious, or worried, or frustrated, or blue.

A Match Made in . . . the Refrigerator?

There's no real harm in finding comfort in a pint of double fudge brownie ice cream—as long as you do it only once in a blue moon. But when you eat to buffer strong negative emotions, to escape reality, or to experience emotional fulfillment, then it begins to disrupt your eating habits.

Emotional eating is cyclical in nature. Suppose you're upset over an argument with your spouse. You turn to food for solace, and you may even feel better for a time. But then guilt, anger, and frustration set in. You're disappointed in yourself for bingeing, and your self-esteem drops. This leads you to isolate yourself from others—and when you do, you feel lonely, bored, and empty. So what do you do? That's right: You eat some more.

This "blue mood, more food" cycle can go on forever. There is one way to stop it, though: Identify and resolve the problem that's driving you to binge in the first place. Breaking patterns of emotional eating will leave you free to experience your true feelings, to more easily reach and maintain a healthy weight, and to truly enjoy food—even an occasional goody—to its fullest.

Food without Guilt

This brings up a very important point: Food is a good thing. After all, you couldn't live without it. You can— and should—find pleasure in it.

"Eating can be a wonderful experience," says Connie Roberts, R.D., manager of nutrition consultation services and wellness programs at Brigham and Women's Hospital in Boston. "Some women think that their food troubles stem from enjoying food too much. The key is to learn to have fun with food, without guilt."

That means—you guessed it—reining in emotion-driven eating. Really, it's much easier than you may think. The following strategies will help you do it.

Take 10. When you get the urge to eat, wait 10 minutes before you head for the fridge. This gives you a little time to regroup and to figure out what may have caused the craving, explains Sandra Campbell, Psy.D., clinical director of the eating disorders program at the Brattleboro Retreat in Vermont. When the 10 minutes are up, you may realize that you no longer want to eat.

Create a diversion. Shift your attention to another, nonfood-related activity. At work, read your mail or flip through the newspaper. At home, polish a pair of shoes or repot your favorite fern. Do one small thing—but make it an activity that can compete with eating. (In other words, cleaning the oven probably won't cut it.)

Invest a few minutes of your time to come up with a list of alternative activities. Post it on your refrigerator at home or tack it to your calendar at work. Then when you're in the mood for food, check your list and see what you could do instead.

Select your snack. You've delayed, you've distracted, and you still feel the need to eat. Go ahead—but think about what you really want, suggests Susan Moore, R.D., program manager and senior nutritionist in the George Washington University Obesity Management Program in Washington, D.C. Are you after a specific taste? Or are you looking for a food that can fill you up? Besides helping you to make more healthful choices, this tactic reminds you that you—not your craving—are controlling the situation.

Do what feels good. From a nutrition standpoint, it's better to tame your craving with, say, a bagel rather than a candy bar. But sometimes a bagel just won't do. On occasions when you absolutely, positively have to have a goody, help yourself—but watch the portion size.

"I have patients practice buying just one chocolate truffle and enjoying it to the utmost," Roberts says. The point is to not deny yourself the one food that you really want. If you do, you may end up consuming more fat and calories by trying to satisfy your craving with something else.

Take your time. These days, many of us eat with a fork in one hand and a pen, a newspaper, or a remote

Feel-Good Foods

Sweets and other high-fat foods provide a quick fix for a foul mood. Unfortunately, while their effects don't last, the pounds they pack on do.

The following chart can help you choose the right food to counterbalance your mood, according to Cheryl Hartsough, R.D., director of wellness and health programs at The Aspen Club in Colorado.

When You Feel . . .	Avoid . . .	Eat . . .
Depressed	Cake, ice cream, pastries	Whole-grain entrées such as pasta primavera or rice and beans
Sleepy and lethargic	Sweets, pizza, high-fat foods	Low-fat, high-protein foods such as broiled or baked fish, veal, poultry, nonfat or low-fat cheese, and egg-white omelets
Tense, anxious, or stressed	Chocolate, cake, ice cream	Fresh fruit, dried fruit, pasta, whole-grain bread, baked potato, rice, vegetables

control in the other. We pay little attention to the process of eating—and we eat too much as a result.

Consume your food slowly and mindfully. Focus on each forkful. By "tuning in" in this way, you're less likely to overeat, explains Barbara Dickinson, R.D., director of nutrition at the weight-management center at Loma Linda University in California and co-leader of the women and food support group.

Conserve calories. So you've indulged a craving. That doesn't mean you've ditched your diet for the entire day. Just figure out how many extra calories you consumed, then perform a little nip-and-tuck on the rest of your meals to compensate. If you ate a 250-calorie candy bar in the afternoon, forgo the dressing on your salad and the butter on your bread at dinner.

Re-engineer your eating environment. Go through all the places you store food, and trade in the high-fat, high-calorie fare for more wholesome selections, suggests Chris Rosenbloom, R.D., Ph.D., associate professor in the department of nutrition and dietetics at Georgia State University in Atlanta and a spokesperson for the American Dietetic Association. "If you open the refrigerator and see a bowl of sliced peaches, chances are, you'll try them," she says.

Lean toward lean. As you restock, keep your eye on the fat content of the foods you choose. Besides the fact that low-fat foods are healthier for you, they can actually help you beat the blues.

When 555 people reduced their dietary fat intakes to 20 percent of calories for a year, they reported feeling less depressed and anxious and more vigorous than they did in the days when they thought chocolate chip cookie dough was a viable dinner option. Should you aim that low? That depends on your individual health status. Generally, though, it's a good idea to limit your dietary fat intake to 25 percent of calories.

Listen to the buzz on Bs. Also lay in a plentiful supply of foods rich in the B-complex vitamins, particularly vitamin B_6, folate, and vitamin B_{12}. This trio is crucial for sound mental health, Somer says. "Surveys show that many women consume less than the 2 milligrams of vitamin B_6 they need each day," she points out. This may help explain why women experience depression more frequently than men, she adds.

Choose baked potatoes, bananas, and chickpeas for vitamin B_6, and lentils, pinto beans, and spinach for folate. Steamed clams and oysters are among the top sources of vitamin B_{12}.

Keep an eye on omega-3's. Nearly 30 percent of certain nerve cell membranes are made from a type of omega-3 fatty acid. Researchers think that when the membranes run low on this fatty acid, they interfere with nerve transmissions and contribute to emotional distress.

Research suggests that maintaining an adequate supply of omega-3's in your system can help steady your emotions. In one small study of patients with clinical depression, those with the most serious cases also had the lowest levels of omega-3's. In a separate study, Japanese students who took fish-oil supplements—a source of omega-3's—were less likely to exhibit hostility toward others during the pressure-cooker atmosphere at the end of the semester.

To get a healthy dose of omega-3's, eat one or two 3-ounce servings of omega-3–rich fish every week. Among the best sources are salmon, herring, bluefin tuna, and mackerel.

Eat at intervals. Skipping breakfast and skimping

on lunch can leave you hungry, grouchy, and vulnerable to emotional eating. To keep your mood—and your energy level—on a more even keel, plan to eat a small meal at least every 4 hours, Dickinson advises.

Eating on a schedule has another advantage, too. If you find yourself feeling hungry at "odd" times, you can assume that your emotions are doing the talking—not your stomach. Then dig a little deeper to discover what's really behind your urge to eat.

Get your snacks in sync. If you tend to eat because you're bored, plan low-fat, low-calorie, fun snacks for between 3:00 and 4:00 P.M. and 8:00 and 9:00 P.M. According to Roberts, research has shown these to be the times of day when "recreational eating" is most likely to take place.

Anticipate emotional eating. If you know you're going to be in a situation where emotional eating is likely, prepare for it. You may want to cut back your calorie intake a bit to give yourself a little breathing room. (Just remember: Don't skip meals!)

Consider the alternatives. As a long-term goal, explore other coping techniques that don't involve food, says Maria Simonson, Sc.D., Ph.D., professor emeritus and director of the health, weight, and stress clinic at the Johns Hopkins Medical Institutions in Baltimore. Aromatherapy, meditation, yoga, and scores of other self-care options can help you feel better—and perhaps, in turn, eat less.

The Calming Cuisine

How to Beat Stress with Food

S tress? No one has to tell you what it feels like. Heck, you're convinced that if you looked up the word in a dictionary, you'd find a photo of yourself.

When stress sets up shop in our lives, our eating habits suffer—big-time. We tend to skip meals, and when we do eat, we make some less-than-admirable food choices. "People grab whatever they can get their hands on; often that's junk food," says Carla Wolper, R.D., a nutritionist for the obesity research center at St. Luke's–Roosevelt Hospital Center and the center for women's health at Columbia-Presbyterian Medical Center, both in New York City.

The bad part is that this downslide into dietary dereliction happens just as our bodies really need us to feed them well. Stress not only interferes with the absorption of nutrients, it also accelerates their excretion. When its nutrient stores are depleted, it's hard for your body to keep up with the demands that stress places on it. Over time, this can take a toll on your health.

But it doesn't have to be that way. In fact, the latest research shows that eating more of some foods and less of others can actually stymie the effects of stress. Adjusting your diet can produce chemical changes in your brain and body that leave you feeling calmer, more relaxed, and ready to face whatever the world throws your way.

Nutritional Antidotes for Stress

To keep your energy and emotions on an even keel and to safeguard your health in the process, give these de-stressing dietary strategies a try.

Calm with carbs. Complex carbohydrates—found in abundance in foods such as pasta, bagels, and baked potatoes—stimulate production of a brain chemical called serotonin. Serotonin mellows your mood, so you feel less tense and anxious and more calm and relaxed. Even better, research has shown that serotonin acts as something of a natural appetite suppressant. The higher your level of serotonin, the less you'll be tempted to overeat.

You can use complex carbohydrates to your advantage when you know you're going to be faced with a stressful task. Suppose you have to make a major presentation at work. Help yourself to some complex carbs about a half-hour before showtime, suggests Judith Wurtman, Ph.D., nutrition research scientist at the Massachusetts Institute of Technology in Cambridge and author of *Managing Your Mind and Mood through Food*. You'll need to eat about 1½ ounces of carbohydrates—2 cups of Cheerios, for example—in order to experience the tranquilizing effects, Dr. Wurtman says.

Be sugar-free. Don't let sugar's status as a simple carbohydrate fool you. It doesn't affect your body in the same way that some of its complex cousins do. Sugar gets absorbed from your bloodstream into cells quite quickly, giving you an almost instantaneous energy boost. Consequently, your blood sugar level can go for a roller-coaster ride, rising and then falling. And that can leave you moody and miserable.

Befriend B$_6$. In a study at the Jean Mayer USDA Human Nutrition Research Center on Aging at Tufts University in Boston, a group of volunteers experienced increases in irritability and tension when their diets ran low on vitamin B$_6$. Researchers suspect that there's a link between B$_6$ and dopamine, a brain chemical that at moderate levels is associated with feeling good. When you don't get enough B$_6$, your dopamine supply is depleted, and you end up being even more susceptible to the effects of stress.

You can boost your B$_6$ intake by choosing foods such as bananas, potatoes, and prunes. One banana, for instance, supplies about 0.7 milligram of B$_6$. If that seems low, keep in mind that the Daily Value for B$_6$ is just 2 milligrams.

Arm yourself with antioxidants. Research has proven that stress causes your body to step up its production of free radicals, destructive molecules that damage healthy tissue and weaken the immune system. This, in turn, can pave the way for serious ailments such as heart disease and some cancers.

The antioxidant nutrients—beta-carotene and vitamins C and E—intervene in that process, neutralizing the free radicals and pulling the plug on their dirty work. In times of stress, you can do your health a favor by eating lots of antioxidant-rich foods as well as by taking an antioxidant-rich multivitamin/mineral supplement, says Elizabeth Somer, R.D., author of *Nutrition for Women* and *Food and Mood*. Carrots, broccoli, and sweet potatoes offer abundant supplies of beta-carotene. For vitamin C, choose oranges, ki-wifruit, tomatoes, and sweet red peppers. Vitamin E is plentiful in wheat germ and vegetable oils. (Just be sure to avoid oils that contain high amounts of saturated fat, such as coconut and palm.)

The Right Food at the Right Time

Anti-stress eating is as much a matter of when you eat as what you eat.

Fuel up first thing. You should make a point of eating breakfast every day. But on high-stress days, your morning meal takes on special significance. The right mix of foods can give you an energy boost that will sustain you at least until noon. The following tempting A.M. menu is recommended by Georgia Hodgkin, R.D., Ed.D., associate professor in the department of nutrition and dietetics at Loma Linda University in California: high-fiber, low-sugar cereal with skim milk; a bagel, an English muffin, or a slice of toast with a tablespoon of peanut butter or nonfat cream cheese; and fruit or fruit juice.

Choose a light lunch. A heavy, high-fat noon-time meal can leave you fatigued and lethargic—not what you want when you have an audience with the boss or a bank loan officer at 2:00 P.M. Eating that way at dinner is no better. Fat takes a long time to digest, and that can prevent you from getting a good night's sleep just when you need it most.

Stick with leaner, lighter fare for your midday and evening repasts. In fact, some experts recommend limiting your total daily fat intake to no more than 25 percent of calories.

Downsize your meals. Some experts believe that in times of stress, we're better off consuming mini-

(continued on page 238)

Eat Away At Stress

Now you know why they call it the daily grind: It sure has made mincemeat out of you. You just can't wait to slip into your comfiest sweats and curl up on the sofa with a nice big bowl of ice cream. Or mashed potatoes with butter. Or macaroni and cheese. These are classic comfort foods that many people turn to in times of stress.

While they sure taste good going down, they're not exactly nutrient-dense—with the exception of fat, of course. And because stress depletes your body of key vitamins and minerals to begin with, you run the risk of putting yourself in the red, nutrition-wise.

There are healthier alternatives. Take a look at the following chart.

Food	Portion	Nutrients
Apple (with skin)	1 (5 oz)	Vitamin C, fiber
Apricots	3 (3.5 oz total)	Beta-carotene, vitamin C
Banana	1 (4 oz)	Vitamin B_6, vitamin C, fiber
Beet greens, boiled	½ cup	Beta-carotene, vitamin C, riboflavin, magnesium
Cabbage, Chinese, shredded, boiled	½ cup	Beta-carotene, vitamin B_6, vitamin C

Food	Portion	Nutrients
Cantaloupe, cubed	1 cup	Beta-carotene, vitamin C
Carrot	1 (2½ oz)	Beta-carotene, vitamin C, fiber
Cauliflower	3 florets (2 oz total)	Vitamin C
Nectarine	1 (5 oz)	Beta-carotene, vitamin C, fiber
Peas, green, boiled	½ cup	Thiamin, folate, vitamin C, fiber
Pineapple, cubed	1 cup	Vitamin C, fiber
Potato, boiled	1 (5 oz)	Vitamin B_6, vitamin C, fiber
Sweet potato, baked	1 (4 oz)	Beta-carotene, vitamin B_6, vitamin C, fiber
Swiss chard, chopped, boiled	½ cup	Beta-carotene, vitamin C, fiber, magnesium, iron
Tomato	1 (4 oz)	Beta-carotene, vitamin C, fiber

meals instead of the standard three squares. This is because eating small portions more often keeps blood sugar levels on a more even keel. In fact, research has shown that when you go for more than 4 hours without eating, your blood sugar level drops low enough to cause fatigue. And while a big meal can leave you feeling sluggish, a mini-meal won't, says Tammy Baker, R.D., a nutritionist in Scottsdale, Arizona, and a spokesperson for the American Dietetic Association.

How do you make the switch to mini-meals? Perhaps the easiest way, according to Elizabeth A. Brown, R.D., nutritionist and weight-control specialist at the Lehigh Valley Hospital Center for Health Promotion and Disease Prevention in Allentown, Pennsylvania, is to divide each of your usual big meals into two smaller ones, then spread them out so that you're eating every 3 to 4 hours.

Chocoholics Anonymous

What You Crave and Why

So just how serious is the love affair between people and chocolate?

Well, in one survey, half of those surveyed said that they would prefer eating chocolate to having sex—which should give their amorous spouses something to think about the next time Valentine's Day rolls around.

Sure, other sweets flirt with our senses, but chocolate has the power to make so many people swoon, particularly women. "Often women tell me that chocolate is the one thing they can count on to give them pleasure whenever they want it," says Anne Kearney-Cooke, Ph.D., director of the Cincinnati Psychotherapy Institute. By one estimate, chocolate accounts for 68 percent of cravings among women.

For all its sweetness, chocolate has its dark side—nutritionally speaking, anyway. It doesn't offer much in the way of nutrients: It has lots of calories and saturated fat and few vitamins and minerals. Every health-conscious bone in your body may tell you to avoid the stuff. Still, when the urge to indulge strikes, you may find it almost impossible to resist.

You can conquer that craving without blowing your

healthy eating habits. And you don't necessarily have to break off your relationship with chocolate to do it.

Sweet Emotions

One survey found that 97 percent of us get a yen for some food or another from time to time. What could possibly make you want a food so badly that you would walk a mile uphill in a raging snowstorm to get it?

Craving may be your body's way of persuading you to replenish its supply of certain substances. We sometimes yearn for sweet, fatty foods such as chocolate when we're running low on endorphins, "feel-good" brain chemicals that boost mood, according to Debra Waterhouse, R.D., author of *Outsmarting the Female Fat Cell* and *Why Women Need Chocolate*. Feed the craving, and your endorphins bounce back, improving your mood, she explains.

Other scientific explanations for chocolate cravings abound. Some experts say that chocolate elevates levels of a soothing brain chemical called serotonin. Others contend that it compensates for a magnesium deficit.

Then again, maybe we want chocolate simply because it tastes so darn good.

Ride the Crave Wave

Chocolate, in itself, really isn't all bad. In fact, there is tantalizing evidence that it may actually have some health *benefits*. Scientists at the University of California, Davis, discovered that chocolate contains flavonoids—the same compounds that give red wine its heart disease–defying punch.

Problems arise when chocolate becomes a dietary staple, crowding out other, more nutritious foods. That's when the fat and calories start adding up.

So how do you balance your healthy eating habits with the overwhelming urge to splurge? Score a craving coup with these smart strategies.

Tune in to your cues. This may be the most important piece of advice, not just for managing your cravings but for managing your entire diet. You need to distinguish between a real, physical need for a food and a desire to eat that's triggered by some external factor—perhaps the sight or smell of a food.

Count on your stomach, your hormones, and your brain chemicals to steer you in the right direction. They'll lay low as long as your body is properly fed. And when it's not, they'll speak up. Your stomach will growl, and your hormones and brain chemicals will place the order: "Send us something sweet!"

Wait it out. When a craving strikes, don't give in to it right away. Instead, try to put off eating for 10 minutes or so. That's about how long it takes for a craving to run its course.

We know that 10 minutes can seem like an eternity when you're convinced that a certain candy bar is calling your name. So distract yourself by taking a walk.

Fool it with fruit. If you have a hankering for something sweet, a piece of fresh fruit just might fill the bill. And it won't send your blood sugar on a roller-coaster ride like chocolate and other sweets can. When that happens, your craving may be intensified.

Stay low. A low-fat or nonfat treat can tame your craving without guilt. For instance, when nothing but chocolate will do, fix yourself a cup of homemade cocoa made with low-fat (1 percent) milk. Two tablespoons of the cocoa powder supply just 1 gram of fat. Or enjoy a "cold fondue" recipe suggested by Elizabeth Somer, R.D., author of *Nutrition for Women* and *Food*

241

and Mood: Serve up 2 cups of cut fresh fruit and ¼ cup of chocolate syrup.

Other saintly skinny selections that may satisfy your chocolate craving include the following:

♦ Entenmann's Light Fudge Brownie—0 grams of fat, 120 calories

♦ Alba Dairy Shake Mix made with skim milk—0 grams of fat, 70 calories

♦ Quaker Chewy Low-Fat Chocolate Chunk Granola Bar—2 grams of fat, 110 calories

♦ SnackWell's Devil's Food Cookie Cakes (2 cookies)—0 grams of fat, 100 calories

Have a little something. Sometimes you can't quiet a chocolate craving with anything less than the real, full-fat, full-calorie thing. When that's the case, do what you have to do. Just keep the portion small, Somer says. One-half ounce—about equal to three chocolate kisses—should do the trick. You'll get about 75 calories and almost 5 grams of fat.

If you can, eat your chocolate with a meal, Somer adds. That way, you're less likely to overdo than if you have a candy bar and nothing else.

PART 5

Your Guide to Eating Out

Restaurant Rules

Mind Your Menu P's and Q's

According to a National Restaurant Association survey, the average American eats out about four times a week. That's 208 times a year—208 meals in which you put your healthy eating habits on the line.

At home, you control what goes into a dish, how it's prepared, and how much of it you put on your plate. Restaurants, though, are a whole other ball game. You find yourself at the mercy of whoever is wielding the pots and pans in the kitchen. What's more, everything from the menu to the decor entices you with the same subliminal message: "You must be famished. C'mon. Eat up!"

Heeding this call didn't matter so much, say, 20 years ago, when folks dined out less frequently. "But these days, with one-third of our calories coming from foods eaten away from home, what we put in our mouths in restaurants does count," says Jayne Hurley, R.D., senior nutritionist with the Center for Science in the Public Interest, a nonprofit consumer group in Washington, D.C., and a writer for *Nutrition Action Healthletter*.

Unfortunately, while eating out has become at least an every-other-day ritual for many of us, we still tend to think of away-from-home meals as treats. This mind-set leads us to choose foods that have too many calories, too much fat, and too few vitamins and minerals. When we walk into restaurants, it seems, the principles of good nutrition get checked at the door.

Make no mistake: They absolutely do count. But they don't mean that you have to nibble on the cottage-cheese-on-lettuce "diet plate" while your dining companions feast on prime rib. On the contrary, you can order a meal that satisfies your appetite but doesn't fill you with guilt in the process. A little strategizing is the key.

Eating Right Made Easy

You can start planning for your meal long before you even set foot in the restaurant. Here's what the experts recommend.

Preview the menu. Stop by your favorite restaurants as well as any new ones you'd like to try and request copies of their menus. Then keep them at home or in your office, so you can decide what you want to order before you venture out to eat. Choosing your meal ahead of time makes you less likely to succumb to the beckoning sight and scent of other, less nutritious foods.

Save up for a splurge. If you're going out for a special occasion—perhaps a coworker's birthday or your wedding anniversary—and you know you might overindulge, simply "bank" some calories by eating a little bit less at preceding meals, suggests Carole Livingston, author of *I'll Never Be Fat Again*. That way, you can enjoy your food without guilt because you know you haven't blown your calorie budget.

But don't go too far and skip meals. It simply doesn't work. When mealtime finally rolls around, you're famished, and you end up stuffing yourself.

Use your imagination. As part of her premeal preparation, Hope S. Warshaw, R.D., author of *The Restaurant Companion: A Guide to Healthier Eating*

Out, says that she does a mental run-through of what she's going to order. She says it helps her to eat healthfully in restaurants, and she recommends that you do the same.

"Mental imagery is very powerful. When you envision yourself succeeding, it's more likely that you will," agrees Susan Olson, Ph.D., clinical psychologist and weight management consultant in Seattle and author of *Keeping It Off: Winning at Weight Loss*.

Sup solo. Researchers at Georgia State University in Atlanta found that people tend to eat more in the presence of others. In fact, the more dining partners you have, the more food you consume. In the study, eating with one person increased food consumption by 28 percent; with two people, by 41 percent; and with six or more people, by 76 percent. The researchers theorize that having company at mealtime causes you to linger over your food. So eating by yourself may not be a bad idea.

Make the first move. If you do eat with others, try to place your order first. That way, you won't be swayed by everyone else's meal choices.

Be nosy. Don't shy away from grilling your server about various menu items. You have a right to know exactly what it is that you're eating and whether it meets your nutrition standards.

Design your own dish. If you can't find something on the menu that suits you, ask whether the chef can "customize" a meal for you. For instance, you may notice that the restaurant serves pasta as well as a steamed vegetable side dish. Perhaps the chef can combine the two. "Don't be afraid to make special requests," Livingston says. "Often, the better the restaurant, the easier it is to make alternate choices."

(continued on page 250)

Red Light, Green Light

Those fancy-schmancy words and phrases in restaurant menus often reveal a great deal about what's in a dish or how it's prepared. You just have to know how to interpret them.

The following glossary features some key terms that you're likely to come across when you eat out, along with a brief definition of each. Keep in mind that recipes can vary from one restaurant to the next, so it's still a good idea to ask the server about ingredients and cooking methods.

Alfredo: A rich sauce made from a combination of butter, Parmesan cheese, and heavy cream.

Au fromage: The French term for "with cheese."

Au gratin: Refers to a dish that is topped with either cheese or a mixture of bread crumbs and butter, then baked until brown.

Au lait: The French term for "with milk."

Bearnaise: A thick sauce that includes white wine, egg yolks, and butter among its ingredients.

Bisque: A rich soup usually made from pureed seafood and cream.

Bolognese: A sauce that's prepared by sautéing meat (usually ground beef, ham, and/or pork) and vegetables in butter, then adding wine and milk or cream for flavor.

Braised: Indicates that a food is cooked in liquid.

Carbonara: A sauce that lists cream, eggs,

Parmesan cheese, and bacon bits among its ingredients.

Florentine: A term used to refer to a dish that is served or dressed with spinach.

Grilled: Indicates that the food is cooked by setting it on a rack directly over a heat source, allowing the fat to drain away.

Hollandaise: A creamy, rich sauce made from butter, egg yolks, and lemon juice.

Marinara: A tomato-based sauce seasoned with basil, garlic, oregano, and onions.

Poached: Indicates that the food is gently cooked in liquid just below the boiling point.

Primavera: Refers to the use of fresh vegetables in a dish. (Just make sure that they're not coated with a cream sauce.)

Steamed: Indicates that the food is placed on a rack or in a steamer basket over boiling or simmering water in a covered pan.

Stir-fried: Indicates that the food is rapidly cooked in a pan or wok; should use little or no oil.

Sweet-and-sour: A sauce that includes sugar and vinegar among its ingredients for a balance of flavors.

Tempura: Indicates that the dish contains fish or vegetables that have been batter-dipped and deep-fried.

Vinaigrette: An oil-and-vinegar combination used to flavor salads and other cold dishes.

Start with soup. In a study at Johns Hopkins University in Baltimore, people who began a meal with a soup appetizer consumed 25 percent fewer calories over the course of the meal than people who had a cheese-and-crackers appetizer. The researchers theorize that soup fills you up, so you don't feel like eating as much. Just remember to steer clear of any concoctions that begin with the words *Cream of*.

Favor fish. If you can't make up your mind, fish is almost always a smart choice. Besides being low in fat, many varieties—including salmon, mackerel, tuna, and herring—have an abundance of omega-3 fatty acids. Research has shown that omega-3's can improve your cholesterol profile and lower your risk of heart disease.

Of course, fish loses its nutritional value when it's fried or coated with butter, cheese, or tartar sauce. Ask to have yours grilled, broiled, steamed, baked, or blackened, Hurley suggests.

Put side dishes in the spotlight. Who says you have to order an entrée? You can create a perfectly acceptable meal by picking and choosing among side dishes and appetizers. This is an excellent way to increase your intake of grains, vegetables, and fruits, notes Evelyn Tribole, R.D., author of *Healthy Homestyle Cooking* and *Eating on the Run*. Plus, you get to sample a little bit of everything, which makes for a more interesting meal.

Dress yourself. Request that any sauce or salad dressing be served on the side. This allows you to control how much goop goes on your food. In fact, instead of pouring it on, leave it in the container. Lightly dip your fork in the sauce or dressing, then pick up a forkful of food. You get the flavor without a huge dose of fat and calories.

Drown your appetite. Drinking lots of water

throughout a meal can fill you up, so you feel less hungry. Ask your server to bring a bottle of mineral water or a pitcher of tap water to your table, then sip constantly.

Bypass the bar. Drinking and dining don't mix. Besides supplying empty calories, alcoholic beverages also enhance your appetite, causing you to overeat. If you want something bubbly, have a glass of club soda with a twist instead.

Take half home. Ask your server to put half of your meal in a doggie bag before bringing the rest to your table. Then have him keep the bag in the kitchen until you're ready to leave. This tactic should reduce the temptation to try to scarf down the whole thing in one sitting. Even better, you'll have a nice lunch or dinner for the next day.

Finish last. People who have weight problems tend to eat faster than people who don't. So take your time. Eat a portion of your meal, then lay down your fork and wait 10 minutes or so before taking another bite. This technique enables you to savor the entire dining experience—the food and the conversation. And at the end of 10 minutes, you may just find that you're not hungry anymore. If you are, then help yourself to a few more forkfuls.

Ethnic Eating

Best and Worst Restaurant Choices

Where in the world should you go for dinner? Thanks to the proliferation of ethnic eateries in this country, you can treat your tastebuds to authentic Greek souvlakia, Japanese yakitori, or Indian chapati without traveling too far from home. In fact, according to a survey conducted by the National Restaurant Association, 98 percent of restaurants have some sort of ethnic dishes on their menus.

The popularity of ethnic cuisine in the United States shouldn't come as a big surprise. After all, our nation's status as the world's melting pot has bestowed us with a wonderfully diverse culinary heritage. And with a growing public awareness of the link between good nutrition and good health, many folks view ethnic foods as healthful alternatives to hamburgers, hot dogs, and other all-American fare.

"In most ethnic places, you can get a lot more vegetables and grains as well as lighter sauces," notes Aliza Green, a restaurant food consultant in Elkins Park, Pennsylvania, and former chef. "And the more authentic the restaurant, the better."

Still, that doesn't mean that all ethnic dishes are automatically good for you. Intermingled with those veggies and grains may lurk a fair amount of butter, cream, or oil. So you need to exercise some caution when placing your order. Take fettuccine Alfredo, for example, Green says. In some Italian restaurants, it's the most frequently ordered entrée. But it's loaded with cream and butter. (The fat content of the dish is so high that some nutritionists darkly dub it "heart attack on a plate.")

You can avoid nutrition traps. You just have to know what to look for. Join us on a culinary world tour, exploring 11 of the best-known and best-loved ethnic cuisines. We asked a number of nutrition authorities to point out which foods to choose and which to avoid, so you can put together a meal that satisfies your nutrition sense and pleases your palate. Consider what follows your passport to healthy ethnic eating.

Welcome to the World's Fare

First, familiarize yourself with the following ethnic-eating ground rules. They apply to any cuisine, from French to Mexican.

Speak up. Even the most detailed menu descriptions don't always tell the whole story. Ask questions about the ingredients and cooking methods used to prepare a particular dish. Otherwise, you may end up getting more fat and calories than you bargained for. If an ingredient or the cooking method doesn't quite suit you, find out if it can be changed. Most chefs are willing to do what it takes to make their patrons happy.

Show the entrée the exit. Order a couple of appetizers rather than a single entrée. This strategy is especially good with Indian, Thai, and Chinese foods. It saves you from huge main-dish portions and allows you to experience the different tastes and textures characteristic of the cuisine. Be careful, though: Since appetizers are often finger foods, you can easily eat too much by picking and nibbling your way through the meal.

Order for two. You can trim down an oversize portion by splitting an entrée with a companion, says Hope S. Warshaw, R.D., author of *The Restaurant Companion: A Guide to Healthier Eating Out.* "In Asian restaurants, you typically split things," Warshaw points out. "I do this all the time. At one typical restaurant meal, for example, three of us shared two different dishes."

Italian: Pasta Perfect

You don't have to travel to Rome to do as the Romans do—at least not when it comes to eating. By one estimate, as many as two-thirds of all restaurants in the United States offer Italian dishes. Indeed, more people order Italian than any other type of food, making it the most popular ethnic cuisine in this country.

For the nutrition-conscious, a plate of pasta makes a delicious meal, without a lot of fat. The vast majority of pasta dishes get no more than 30 percent of calories from fat and no more than 10 percent of calories from saturated fat.

But authentic Italian cuisine is much more than just pasta. Vegetable and bean dishes are quite common, too. In fact, the people of southern Italy follow what many nutritionists consider to be the healthiest diet in the world: the Mediterranean diet, which is characterized by lots of grains and produce, little meat, and olive oil instead of butter.

Travel to the northern part of the country, and you'll discover an entirely different version of Italian cuisine. There, the more beef, butter, and cream in a dish, the better folks seem to like it.

This, unfortunately, is the cooking style that most restaurants on this side of the Atlantic emulate. We favor fettuccine Alfredo, lasagna, and anything parmigiana—which, naturally, are loaded with calories and fat.

"Italian food is simple. The secret is the pasta," says Jayne Hurley, R.D., senior nutritionist with the Center for Science in the Public Interest, a nonprofit consumer group in Washington, D.C., and a writer for *Nutrition Action Healthletter*. "As long as you get spaghetti or linguine, you can top it with tomato sauce, marinara sauce, red or white clam sauce, meat sauce, even meatballs, and you're practically guaranteed a lower-fat meal."

Become a bean counter. Beans figure prominently in authentic Italian cuisine. Pasta e fagioli, for instance, is a soup that combines pasta and white beans (or *fagioli*, in Italian). Minestrone is similar, except that the cook throws vegetables into the mix. Take advantage of these dishes to increase your daily fiber intake.

Order goodness by the slice. And you thought pizza was junk food? Consider this: The crust supplies carbohydrates; the cheese, protein and calcium; and the sauce and vegetables, vitamins A and C. Skip the meat toppings, and you have a healthful food that gets a respectable 25 to 30 percent of its calories from fat.

Bag the garlic bread. Yes, it's bread, and you're supposed to eat bread. But toasted garlic bread is soaked in oil or butter. Request plain Italian bread instead, and if you must have something on it, spread your slice with just the thinnest smear of butter.

Be anti-antipasto. Beware the antipasto dishes that include olives, cheeses, and smoked meats. Besides supplying fat and sodium that you don't need, these foods jack up the calorie content of your meal. If you want something to nibble on, order a vegetable antipasto with grilled mushrooms, roasted peppers, zucchini, and caponata (a Sicilian relish).

Help Yourself To . . .

♦ Any dish described as marsala (broth-based and cooked with wine)

♦ Chicken cacciatore

♦ Cioppino (a fish stew)

♦ Marinara, pizzaola, and other meatless, tomato-based sauces

♦ Pasta primavera (as long as it doesn't have a cream or butter sauce)

Hands Off . . .

♦ Any cheese-filled pasta such as cannelloni, lasagna, and ravioli

♦ Any sauce labeled "crema" or "fritto"

♦ Fettuccine Alfredo

♦ Risotto (a rice dish made with butter and cheese)

♦ Veal piccata or saltimbocca

Greek: More Than Just Gyros

Greek cuisine has found its niche in, of all places, the shopping mall food court. Should you visit one of these culinary kiosks, you'll most likely find popular specialties such as gyros, moussaka, and baklava. Unfortunately, these foods tend to be less healthy than most Greek dishes. They don't do justice to this Mediterranean cuisine, yet another variation of what nutritionists now recognize as one of the healthiest cuisines in the world.

Like other people who live in countries of the Mediterranean region, Greeks eat an abundance of grains and vegetables. In fact, most of their meals have bread as the centerpiece. Meat—lamb is a favorite—makes an appearance only on special occasions, and fruit is the dessert of choice.

Greek cooking also uses generous amounts of olive oil. While it is pure fat, it's mostly monounsaturated—the kind that can actually lower your cholesterol and reduce your risk of heart disease.

To enjoy a healthful Greek meal, of course, you may have to stray from the dishes that are most familiar to you—the higher-fat offerings that tend to be most pleasing to the American palate. So as you ponder the menu, keep these pointers in mind.

Go for grilled. Grilling is among the healthiest cooking methods, and Greek chefs tend to do a lot of it. So scan the menu for dishes that feature grilled seafood, poultry, meat, or vegetables. Among the favorites are souvlakia, skewered chunks of marinated lamb, sometimes with green peppers, onions, or other vegetables; and shish kebab, skewered chunks of marinated meat or fish and vegetables.

Slim down your salad. A Greek salad makes a great accompaniment to a meal—or a meal in itself. But you may want to order yours without fatty, salty ingredients such as anchovies and kalamata olives. As always, request your dressing on the side.

Be cautious with cheese. Feta, a classic Greek cheese, has a lot of fat and a lot of salt—mainly because it's preserved in brine. And the popular appetizer saganaki is actually fried kasseri cheese that some restaurants soak in brandy, then serve flambéed. Go easy on both.

Help Yourself To . . .

♦ Baba ghanoush (served as a spread or dip)

♦ Fish baked with plaki sauce (garlic and tomato sauce)

♦ Shish kebab

♦ Souvlakia

♦ Tabbouleh (bulgur mixed with chopped tomatoes, parsley, mint, olive oil, and lemon juice)

♦ Torato (a cold soup made with eggplant, peppers, and yogurt)

♦ Tzatziki (a dip or dressing made from yogurt, garlic, and cucumbers)

Hands Off . . .

♦ Avgolemono (a soup or sauce made with chicken broth, egg yolks, and lemon juice)

♦ Baklava and other rich desserts

♦ Falafel (a dish made with deep-fried chickpea croquettes)

♦ Moussaka (a dish made of meat and eggplant, often covered with egg- or cheese-enriched béchamel sauce)

♦ Spanakopita (a vegetable pie made with feta cheese and eggs)

French: Ooh-La-Lunch

Mention French cuisine, and most people envision rich sauces and to-die-for desserts. If this includes you, then you're in for a healthful surprise. French cooking has undergone a makeover of sorts. Cream and butter, once mainstays of French recipes, have all but slipped from view. In their place are fruits, veggies, and other wholesome, garden-fresh ingredients.

In its high-fat heyday, French cuisine had all the makings of a heart attack waiting to happen. In fact, the French still eat about as much saturated fat as we do. So why do they have the second-lowest rate of heart disease in the world?

Experts believe that the answer lies with the red wine they savor with almost every meal. Red wine has an abundant supply of flavonoids, chemical compounds that help keep the heart healthy.

Don't think, though, that washing down your cassoulet with a glass of Beaujolais will somehow neutralize your meal's artery-clogging effects. The best way to make your dining experience a healthful one is to seek out a dish that features low-fat ingredients and is prepared in a low-fat way. As you scan the menu, keep these tips in mind.

Show a sense of style. French cooking consists of several different styles, and some are fattier than others. When a restaurant says it serves haute cuisine or cuisine bourgeois, that's your cue to be on the lookout for dishes prepared with butter, cream, eggs, and other high-fat ingredients. Nouvelle cuisine, on the other hand, favors fresh ingredients and smaller portions. Even healthier is cuisine minceur, a relatively new style that avoids fats and cream. In fact, its name literally means "cuisine of slenderness."

Select skinny sauce. If you're having a dish with a sauce, look for one that is wine-based rather than cream- or butter-based. If you want to try a dish with a heavy sauce, ask the server if you can get an appetizer-size portion.

Help Yourself To . . .

♦ Bouillabaisse (a seafood stew)

♦ Consommé (meat or fish broth)

♦ French bread

♦ Ratatouille (a vegetable dish cooked in olive oil)

♦ Sauces labeled coulis, puree, reduction, or vegetable

♦ Seafood that is poached or steamed

Hands Off . . .

♦ Cassoulet (a classic meat-and-beans dish featuring sausage, pork, and duck or goose)

♦ Dairy-based sauces such as béarnaise and beurre blanc

♦ Pâté

♦ Quiches

♦ Soufflés

♦ Sweetbreads (which are not bread at all, but organ meats)

Chinese: For Healthy Eating, Look to the East

Nutritionists continue to heap praise on the traditional Chinese diet as one of the healthiest in the world. By eating generous portions of rice and vegetables and only the smallest amounts of meat, native Chinese manage to keep their daily fat intakes to about 15 percent of calories. In the United States, our daily fat intake is more than double that amount.

Come to think of it, that may explain why Chinese cuisine puts on a little weight when it crosses the Pacific to our shores. The Americanized version features mounds of meat, deep-fried appetizers, and pools of sodium-charged soy sauce, while rice is relegated to practically garnish status.

Actually, Chinese cooking varies from region to region, and some styles are healthier than others. Most restaurants in this country specialize in Cantonese dishes, which feature roasted and grilled meat, steamed dishes, and mild flavors. Szechuan cooking, on the other hand, features many fried foods and tends to be hot and spicy. And then there are dishes from Shanghai, the coastal regions of the country, where seafood is a staple ingredient.

Generally, authentic Chinese cuisine favors healthful cooking methods, such as stir-frying and steaming. In fact, rather than ordering an entrée off the restaurant menu, you may want to request a simple dish of chicken or shrimp with steamed vegetables. From a nutrition standpoint, it's one of your best bets, and just about any Chinese chef can do a top-notch job of preparing it.

Here are some more strategies to help you enjoy Chinese cuisine at its healthiest.

Broaden your horizons. Traditional Chinese cooking relies heavily on vegetables. You'll get your fair share of the familiar, like broccoli, cabbage, and peppers. But be sure to introduce yourself to some more exotic selections, too—native favorites such as bamboo shoots, lily pods, lotus root, and water chestnuts.

Sample soy foods. Soy has earned superfood status, and for good reason. Research so far has shown that it may not only minimize the physical effects of menopause but may also reduce the risk of breast cancer. If you want to get more soy foods in your diet, here's your opportunity. Soy is a staple in Chinese

261

cooking. In fact, it supplies most of the protein in the Chinese diet. Look for dishes that have a soy product, such as tofu or miso, as an ingredient.

Sip soup. Chinese restaurant menus usually feature a selection of low-fat, flavorful soups. They're perfect to start your meal or as a main dish. What about the eggs in egg drop soup? They do raise the cholesterol content, but not by much. Incidentally, hot-and-sour soup also has an egg base.

Pick up sticks. If you're having Chinese food (or Thai food), try your hand at chopsticks. You say you're not good at using them? That's even better! They slow you down, so you eat less.

Be sodium-sensitive. One item to watch in Chinese cuisine is sodium. Soy sauce, for instance, supplies 343 milligrams per teaspoon. Monosodium glutamate (MSG) also supplies a generous amount of sodium, one-third as much as table salt. But MSG has yet another downside: It has been linked to headaches.

Eschew cashews. Nuts are fat pills. One large, oil-coated cashew carries about 1 gram of fat. Imagine how that adds up when you pour ½ cup of them into an entrée. So tell your server to hold the nuts—or at least cut the amount to 2 to 3 tablespoons, max.

Don't miss tea time. Most Chinese restaurants serve green tea with their meals. By all means, drink up. Green tea is loaded with compounds called polyphenols, which act like disease-fighting antioxidants. In fact, early research suggests that green tea may help protect against certain types of cancer and heart disease. (Be aware, though, that black tea doesn't have the same therapeutic properties.)

Find your fortune. A fortune cookie has just 30 calories and absolutely no fat. When you compare that with other desserts, your future looks healthier already!

Help Yourself To . . .

♦ Hot-and-sour or wonton soup

♦ Rice (brown is best, but white is okay)

♦ Shrimp with garlic sauce

♦ Szechuan shrimp (stir-fried in hot sauce)

♦ Steamed vegetable dumplings

♦ Stir-fried vegetables

Hands Off . . .

♦ Anything crispy or batter-coated (both terms indicate the food has been fried)

♦ Egg foo yong

♦ Egg rolls

♦ Fried rice

♦ Kung pao chicken

♦ Moo shu pork

Japanese: The Other Asian Cuisine

After years in the shadow of Chinese food, Japanese food has at last come into its own in this country. While Japanese restaurants have yet to match the proliferation of their Chinese counterparts, you'll have a much easier time finding one these days.

All we can say is . . . it's about time! Japanese cooking has much to offer, flavor-wise and nutrition-wise. For starters, it can claim one of the lowest fat contents among ethnic cuisines. Most dishes get less than 20 percent of their calories from fat. Grains and vegetables are dietary mainstays, as are seafood and soy. Meat, however, is not. When it is served, the portion is kept small.

The Japanese favor low-fat cooking methods, too, such as broiling, grilling, and steaming. And they use as little oil as possible.

Not sure what to look for on a Japanese menu? Let these tips serve as your guide.

Use your noodles. Rice is a staple of Japanese cuisine. But if you'd like to try something a little different, order a dish made with buckwheat noodles (soba) or wheat noodles (udon). You'll most likely find them in soups or as "beds" on which other foods are served.

Sample sushi. There's more to sushi than just raw fish. It can take many forms. The main ingredient is actually boiled rice flavored with rice vinegar. The rice may be garnished with fish, tofu, or vegetables, then wrapped in thin sheets of seaweed.

Sushi made with raw fish—especially mackerel and tuna—offers a generous dose of heart-healthy omega-3 fatty acids. And since it's uncooked, it has no added fat. (For more information on eating this Japanese delicacy safely, see "Sushi Savvy" on page 266.)

Try your pot luck. Nabemono—which literally means "things in a pot"—is the Japanese version of a one-dish meal. Yosenabe is one kind of nabemono, featuring chicken, seafood, and vegetables in seasoned broth.

Get wise to sodium. Soy sauce, teriyaki sauce, and miso sauce all have very high sodium contents. They're also quite common in Japanese cooking. If you're concerned about your sodium intake, request that the chef prepare the dish without the sauce and ask for low-sodium soy sauce on the side.

Help Yourself To . . .

♦ Any dish described as nimono (simmered), yaki (broiled), or yakimono (grilled)

♦ Chirinabe (a one-dish meal made with fish, tofu, and vegetables)

♦ Shabu-shabu (meats and vegetables cooked in broth)

♦ Tofu and other soy foods

♦ Yakitori (either grilled or broiled chicken)

Hands Off . . .

♦ Any dish described as agemono (deep-fried) or tempura (batter-dipped and deep-fried)

♦ Fish that has been salted, smoked, or pickled

♦ Sukiyaki

Thai: Is It Hot Enough for You?

If you enjoy Chinese or Japanese food, you may want to give Thai a try. Thai cooking stir-fries lots of rice and vegetables, so it can be just as nutritious as the other Asian cuisines. It also makes extensive use of herbs. Recipes often call for tantalizing, aromatic seasonings such as lemongrass, lime leaves, and Thai basil.

Thai food can be a real adventure for your taste-buds. To make sure it's a healthful one, keep these tips in mind.

Keep an eye on coconut. Coconut milk is a staple of Thai cooking. Unfortunately, it can turn an otherwise healthful dish into a fat-laden fiasco. When added to a curry, for example, it can increase the fat content to more than 40 percent of calories.

(continued on page 268)

Sushi Savvy

Time was when people—okay, college frat boys—would swallow live goldfish only on a dare. Now we're *paying* to sit at sushi bars and eat raw fish.

Of course, there's more to sushi bars than raw fish. The word *sushi* actually refers to vinegared rice. Traditionally, the rice is topped with a wide variety of garnishes, such as cooked egg, raw or cooked fish and shellfish, and cucumbers, avocados, and other vegetables. Technically, sliced raw fish is known as sashimi.

Salmon and tuna are the most popular choices at sushi bars, followed by mackerel, shrimp, rockfish, snapper, abalone, and scallops, among others. But not everyone is gaga over raw fish. Like raw beef, pork, or chicken, raw fish may contain harmful bacteria, such as *Listeria monocytogenes*. To prevent contamination, it's important that raw fish be properly handled. And fish sometimes have parasitic worms. To kill these parasites, raw fish needs to be frozen.

Aside from disease-causing bacteria, certain large tropical fish could harbor hazardous and potentially life-threatening toxins. Be aware that if illegally or recreationally harvested, fish like barracuda, red snapper, and Australian coral trout may harbor what is called a ciguatoxin. This problem, however, does not usually occur with commercial products because their distribution is regulated by the industry.

If served in a well-established restaurant and prepared by a qualified, knowledgeable sushi chef who has undergone years of training, sushi can be safe. The chef knows how to buy the right species of fish during the right season and how to prepare it properly. According to Kayo Io, manager of the Fuki-Sushi Restaurant in Palo Alto, California, word of mouth is the best way to find restaurants with top-notch sushi chefs. But for the very best flavor and freshness, it's important that the fish be eaten within 10 to 20 minutes of preparation.

"If you still have a concern about safety, ask the chef if he freezes the fish or buys it frozen," suggests Ann Adams, Ph.D., a research parasitologist specializing in seafood products at the Food and Drug Administration's seafood products research center in Seattle.

Whatever you do, never eat raw salmon that has never been frozen. There's a higher risk that salmon may be infected with parasites than other fish, says Dr. Adams, who tested almost 500 samples of sushi for parasites.

As for benefits, sushi can play a potential role in a healthy diet. Fish in general is low in fat and a good source of minerals. And fish like salmon, mackerel, and tuna supply healthy omega-3 fatty acids.

If you want to try sushi, start out with a light-tasting fish that's not high in oil, such as halibut or snapper, and shellfish such as abalone, shrimp, or scallops before moving on to oilier fish such as yellowtail, tuna, and mackerel.

Be sure to ask your server how various dishes are prepared. The use of coconut milk or cream may not be obvious.

Feel the heat. If you've never tried Thai food, be forewarned: Many dishes are *very* hot.

Help Yourself To . . .

♦ Forest salad

♦ Pad thai (a stir-fried noodle dish)

♦ Sautéed ginger beef or chicken (but request minimal oil)

♦ Soups made with lemongrass

♦ Yum neua (broiled beef with onions)

Hands Off . . .

♦ Anything served with peanut sauce

♦ Hae Kuen (deep-fried prawn cakes)

♦ Hot Thai catfish (fried)

♦ Royal tofu (fried)

♦ Yum koon chaing (a sausage-and-pepper dish)

Indian: A Complex Treat

Traditional Indian recipes bombard the palate with a unique blend of sweet and spicy. Yogurt often shows up in the same ingredients list as curry powder and other smoldering seasonings.

Perhaps the best-known Indian specialty is curry, which actually is a catch-all term for hot, spicy, gravy-based dishes that get their heat from—appropriately enough—curry powder. Curry powder, in turn, is a blend of up to 20 herbs, spices, and seeds, which may include cardamom, cloves, coriander, cumin, and mace. Curried food is often accompanied by chutney, a spicy condiment that combines fruit, vinegar, sugar, and spices.

The traditional Indian diet includes an abundance of grains, beans, and vegetables. Meat and fish are served not as entrées but as ingredients in entrées.

By all accounts, Indian cuisine has the makings of a healthful diet. But it's not without its nutritional danger zones. Use the following strategies to get through the menu maze.

Try tandoori. Tandoori is a cooking method in which foods are baked in a brick-and-clay oven (called a tandoor). Indian chefs often prepare fish and chicken in this way. When you choose a tandoori dish, you can be confident that you're getting something healthy.

Love those loaves. Don't miss the opportunity to try one of the astounding array of Indian breads. Just make sure that it has been baked rather than fried. Among the names to look for are chapati, kulcha, and naan.

Give up ghee. Many Indian dishes are soaked in ghee, which is clarified butter. When used in the preparation of a food, it can raise the fat content to 50 percent of calories.

Coconut oil, another staple, also has a mean streak. It contains mostly saturated fat—the unhealthy kind.

So ask your server how the dish you'd like to order is prepared. If he mentions either of these ingredients, request that the chef use a lighter cooking oil.

Help Yourself To . . .

♦ Any dish marinated in yogurt

♦ Dal (a spicy dish made with lentils)

♦ Karhi (chickpea soup)

- Khur (a dessert made with milk and rice)
- Mulligatawny (a kind of lentil soup)

Hands Off . . .

- Any dish referred to as kandhari, korma, or malai (indicating that coconut or cream is an ingredient)
- Fried breads such as paratha and poori
- Pakora (deep-fried breads and vegetables)
- Samosa (a fried pastry sometimes stuffed with vegetables or meat)

Cajun: Nice and Spicy

Red-hot spices are the cornerstone of this style of cooking, which got its start on the Louisiana coast. Chefs describe it as a hybrid of French and Creole cuisines. You'll find a lot of seafood on Cajun restaurant menus. It often shows up as an ingredient in a classic Cajun specialty, jambalaya. But Cajun cooking has other traditions that aren't quite so healthy. As you peruse the menu, keep the following in mind.

Find out about fat. With its generous use of seafood, vegetables, and rice, Cajun cooking seems like the nutrition-conscious person's dream. But dig a little deeper, and you'll discover that it uses lots of animal fat, especially pork fat. This is why it's so important to ask your server how a dish is prepared before ordering.

Help Yourself To . . .

- Blackened fish or chicken (heavily seasoned and cooked quickly with little oil)
- Greens, such as kale and okra
- Jambalaya, made without high-fat ingredients such as pork and sausage

- Seafood gumbo
- Shrimp Creole

Hands Off . . .

- Andouille, boudin, and other sausage dishes
- Dirty rice (fried rice mixed with fatty meats)
- Etouffée, a crawfish-and-vegetable stew with a roux base (roux is a combination of flour and fat)
- Hush puppies (deep-fried dumplings)
- Mud pie

Caribbean: Paradise for the Palate

Envision yourself on a tropical island. Then look around. By the roadside, the trees burst with bananas, papayas, avocados, mangoes, oranges, and pineapples—all staples of the Caribbean. And chili bushes stand laden with their pungent fruit—the secret to the special spiciness of many of the islands' best-loved dishes.

In many ways, Caribbean cooking defies categorization. It boasts an array of ethnic influences because people from all over the world—France, Spain, England, Africa, China, India, and Portugal—settled on the islands and brought their native cuisines with them. "Then as people moved around the islands and cultures intermingled, new dishes emerged," explains Donna Morton de Souza, R.D., a nutritionist in Miami and former corporate dietitian for Royal Caribbean International.

Still, de Souza says, there is common ground in Caribbean cooking. Exotic fruits and chili peppers are staple ingredients, as are nutmeg, ginger, and curry spices. You'll notice some bean dishes on menus, too—in fact, black bean soup is considered an island specialty.

271

Because Caribbean cuisine has such a diverse heritage, you may find that restaurants differ in the dishes they serve. But these general guidelines can help you know what to look for.

Try something new. Take advantage of the opportunity to sample some of the Caribbean's exotic native produce. Look for dishes prepared with callaloo, a leafy green that's similar to kale; chayote, a fruit that looks something like an overgrown pear; or breadfruit, a versatile fruit distinguished by its bumpy green skin.

Be careful with coconut. Many Caribbean recipes call for either the meat or the milk of the coconut, or (like Indian or Thai cuisine) they're cooked in coconut oil, de Souza says. But like any other nut, coconut has an abundance of fat—most of it the heart-unhealthy saturated kind. Try to steer clear of dishes that have any form of coconut as an ingredient. If you aren't sure, ask.

Forget fried fare. Frying seems to be the cooking method of choice for many Caribbean dishes. "Take fritters, which are a popular appetizer," de Souza says. "They're made with healthy ingredients, like chickpeas or fish, but then they're deep-fried." Other common deep-fried specialties include codfish cakes, plantain chips, and shrimp with anchovy stuffing.

Pare the portion. "A restaurant may serve a meal a little differently, but when I ate on the islands, I remember getting a heaping plate of food," de Souza says. "It had a little bit of everything." Since most restaurants are given to oversize portions to begin with, you may want to consider sharing a meal with your dining companion—or if not, just take home the extra.

272

Help Yourself To . . .

♦ Black bean soup

♦ Broiled or grilled seafood

♦ Jerk chicken ("jerk" refers to a seasoning blend usually made from chili peppers, garlic, onions, thyme, and spices)

Hands Off . . .

♦ Anything fried

♦ Anything made with coconut, coconut milk, or coconut oil

♦ Baked papaya with meat filling

♦ Blood sausage

♦ Pepper pot

Mexican: Better Run for the Border

Authentic Mexican cuisine bears little resemblance, nutrition-wise, to the Americanized stuff served in most restaurants. The Mexican people tend to follow a healthy high-carbohydrate, low-fat diet with lots of grains and beans and moderate amounts of meat. They use generous amounts of spices to flavor their foods and seldom cook in oil.

When the cuisine migrated across the border, something definitely got lost in the translation of the recipes. Our version of Mexican features gobs of high-fat cheese and sour cream, which you'd be hard-pressed to find south of the border. Everything, it seems, gets soaked in oil and deep-fried. And shredded iceberg lettuce doesn't really count as a nutritious vegetable.

In fact, when the *Nutrition Action Healthletter*

analyzed 15 popular dishes at 19 midpriced Mexican restaurants, only one—chicken fajitas—got less than 30 percent of calories from fat. Most of the meals, which came with accompaniments such as refried beans and guacamole, provided an entire day's allotment of fat in one sitting.

Thankfully, some Mexican restaurants have begun overhauling their menus to offer healthier, more authentic selections. For instance, two of the country's largest Mexican restaurant chains—Chi-Chi's and El Torito—have trimmed the fat from some of their old recipes and developed new, leaner entrées for their health-conscious patrons.

If you can, order à la carte rather than a full dinner. That way, you can bypass all the high-fat, high-calorie trimmings that come on the plate. Here are some more strategies for keeping your Mexican meal nutritious and delicious.

Veg out. Traditional Mexican cooking features an array of exotic, flavorful produce. Look for dishes that contain nopales (cactus leaves), which taste like slightly tart green beans; jícama, a turniplike root vegetable with a nutty flavor; and tomatillos, which look like small green tomatoes but taste like a combination of lemons, apples, and herbs.

Say *si* to salsa. According to the people who keep track of such things, Americans now spend more money on salsa than on ketchup. This condiment—a mix of tomatoes, onions, chilies, and herbs—has practically no fat and supplies generous doses of vitamins A and C to boot. Use it instead of sour cream, cheese, and guacamole to give your meal a burst of flavor.

Skimp on chips. Fifty chips in that complimentary basket of tortilla chips that the server just set under your nose contain more than three-quarters of your fat allotment for the entire day. If you're not careful, they'll disappear before you even crack open the menu.

To limit your chip consumption, decide up front how many you want to eat. Then take that number out of the basket and move the rest out of reach. Even better, have the server return the basket to the kitchen.

Reject refried beans. Unlike many of the canned refried beans that you buy in the supermarket, the restaurant version is usually prepared in lard—sometimes with bacon and cheese added to the mix. A ¾-cup serving supplies a whopping one-third of your daily allotment of saturated fat.

Come out of your shell. If you order a taco salad, resist the temptation to nibble on the tortilla shell that it's served in. And watch out for high-fat toppings, too—black olives, cheese, sour cream, guacamole, and the like.

Help Yourself To . . .

♦ Bean enchiladas

♦ Black bean soup and gazpacho soup

♦ Chicken soft tacos

♦ Fajitas

♦ Seafood prepared Veracruz-style (cooked in an herbed tomato sauce)

♦ Seviche (fish marinated in lime juice)

Hands Off . . .

♦ Chilies rellenos (deep-fried, cheese-stuffed chilies)

♦ Chimichanga

♦ Chorizo (a spicy pork sausage)

- ◆ Flautas (corn tortillas rolled around a meat or poultry filling, then deep-fried)
- ◆ Quesadillas
- ◆ Taquitos (fried)

American Steakhouses: Here's the Beef

In no way does the proliferation of ethnic restaurants suggest that typical American food is on the endangered species list for the food chain. Rather, American food has become yet another ethnic cuisine from which to choose. And nothing captures the essence of the typical American diet like the steakhouse does. Everything comes in one size: big. Make that really big. If that slab of red meat isn't the same circumference as your plate, why, it has no right to be calling itself a steak.

"Steakhouses are known for huge, huge servings," agrees Liz Applegate, Ph.D., a nutrition lecturer at the University of California, Davis, and author of *Power Foods*. When you eat a typical steak, you're getting two or three times—if not four or five times—as much protein as you should be getting.

But red meat does have its virtues. Steak, in particular, is a great source of zinc and a good source of iron and other trace minerals that women tend to run low on. "So it's an item that can be had in the diet," Dr. Applegate says. "The motto here is moderation."

The following tips can help you round up a healthy steakhouse feast.

Skimp on size. If you want steak, order the smallest one on the menu, suggests Evelyn Tribole, R.D., author of *Healthy Homestyle Cooking* and *Eating on the Run*. "Believe me, that is still bigger than you might think."

Mull over the menu. You don't have to order steak just because you're at a steakhouse. The restaurant may offer other entrées, such as shish kebabs or stir-fries, that use meat as an ingredient rather than as the centerpiece of the meal.

Leave the fat behind. If you do order a steak, be sure to trim off all the visible fat before you dig in. This reduces the fat content of your meal a little more.

Choose bird over beef. You might also discover a poultry dish or two on the menu. Poultry, of course, generally has less fat than red meat, and even within the poultry section of the menu, some entrées are healthier than others. Chicken breast, for example, has less saturated fat and cholesterol than chicken legs or wings—especially Buffalo wings. You can spare yourself even more fat grams by removing the skin.

Help Yourself To . . .

♦ Sirloin cuts

♦ Tenderloin cuts, such as filet mignon

Hands Off . . .

♦ Anything with "rib" in the name, such as prime rib, rib-eye, and spareribs

Eating in the Fast Lane

Your Guide to Fast-Food Places

Until about 50 years ago, "fast food" pretty much referred to anything that could outrun a hungry hunter. Then two brothers by the name of McDonald got an idea: Why not run hamburger stands on the same principles of mass production that work so well for manufacturers?

To say their idea caught on is an understatement. Indeed, fast food has become a staple in the typical American diet. At least one survey has shown that 44 percent of us eat in fast-food restaurants at least once a week, making a substantial contribution to the estimated $100 billion the fast-food industry rakes in each year.

Why the love affair with no-frills fare? Convenience is a big factor. And of course, the food does come cheap. The trouble is that you may pay for it in terms of your good health. Many menu mainstays have questionable nutritional profiles, supplying way too much of some nutrients and way too little of others. For instance, most fast-food items get between 40 and 50 percent of their calories from fat. And we all know what kind of damage excessive dietary fat can do to our hearts and our waistlines.

Now none of this means that fast food has no place in a healthy diet. The trick is to make it an occasional treat—and to choose your meal wisely.

Menu Moxie

Contemplating a meal at Bubba's Burger Barn? You can pick up something reasonably healthful—if you know what to look for on the menu. Here's what the experts recommend.

Look at the big picture. As you decide what to order, consider what you've eaten earlier in the day and what you plan to eat later on. Try to strike a nutritional balance with your food choices. And don't forget to round out your meal with add-ons that are a little more nutrient-dense—like a side salad, a piece of fruit, or a carton of skim or low-fat (1 percent) milk.

Select the right size. Sure, those oversize sandwiches, fries, and drinks can save you a few cents. But boy, oh boy, can they tax you nutrition-wise. "Stay away from anything called jumbo, giant, supersize, or colossal," says Jayne Hurley, R.D., senior nutritionist with the Center for Science in the Public Interest, a nonprofit consumer group in Washington, D.C., and a writer for *Nutrition Action Healthletter*. "That's generally a dead giveaway that a food is loaded with calories and fat."

Forget the fried stuff. Stick with sandwiches that are grilled, broiled, or roasted. And while you're at it, tell the person behind the counter to hold the cheese, mayonnaise, "special sauce," and other high-fat goop.

Build a better burger. When you have a hankering for some ground round, select the smallest hamburger on the menu, Hurley suggests. Then dress it up with lettuce, tomatoes, and dollops of ketchup and mustard. Again, try to skip the special sauce—but if you can't bear to taste your burger without it, at least get it on the side, so you have more control over how much you consume, she says.

Make spuds your buds. "People think of French fries as a side dish, but they're really not," Hurley says. "Eating fries is like eating a whole other sandwich." A large order of fries supplies as many calories and as much fat as a McDonald's Quarter Pounder.

Instead, choose a baked potato. It has no fat, no cholesterol, just a smidgen of sodium, and healthy doses of fiber, vitamin C, and other nutrients to boot. For toppings, try broccoli, salsa, or cottage cheese rather than the usual butter or sour cream.

Sip smart. Wash down your meal with juice or skim or low-fat milk. Both supply valuable vitamins and minerals, and their flavors nicely complement just about any food. Soda can be okay, too. Just remember that in terms of nutrition, it doesn't hold a candle to juice or milk.

All in the Family

Your Take-the-Kids-Out Survival Guide

It's Friday night at your family's favorite burger palace, and you've just eaten an entire weekend's fat intake in one hour—the proof still shines on your hands. You leave the restaurant feeling bloated, blaming the kids for insisting on coming here, the waitress for taking so long to clear your plate, and the restaurant for blatantly exposing you to the triple-decker cheeseburger photo in the first place.

How can you defend yourself against the onslaught of complimentary chips, monster burgers, and mocha mud pies when you take the kids or grandkids to the local family restaurant?

Starting It Off Right

You haven't finished scooting into the booth and already you're greeted by a basket of free chips and a list of must-try appetizers. Here's how to keep seemingly harmless starters from undermining your efforts.

Simplify your drinks. Craving that fruity non-alcoholic umbrella drink? Better not, says Jane Ziegler, R.D., program coordinator for the Allen Center for Nutrition at Cedar Crest College in Allentown, Pennsylvania. "Specialty drinks have lots of sugar, and they may have cream, whole milk, or ice cream to make them creamy." Let the kids get them and have one sip.

Skip the appetizers. "Appetizers to me are a real danger zone. The meal is usually more than most people can handle anyway, plus appetizers are often high-fat foods," says Ziegler. How high-fat? Well, according to a study by the Center for Science in the Public Interest, which looked at dinner houses across the country, it'll cost you 48 grams of fat for an average order of 12 Buffalo wings, 51 grams of fat for 9 fried mozzarella sticks, and a whopping 79 grams of fat for an 8-piece order of potato skins—and that's not including sour cream.

Start your salad sooner. The kids won, so now you're staring down potato skins. Solution? "Ask that your salad be served immediately," suggests Ziegler. "And try to get to the restaurant at a time when the wait for your entrée won't be long."

Sidestepping Entrée Traps

You know the rule, but you still spend the first half-hour rehearsing it in your head: "Fried—bad; grilled—good." Still, there's a lot on the menu to consider.

Familiarize yourself with these common dinner-house traps before the waiter with the two-tone hair sells you on the quesadilla.

Plan ahead. Don't jump headfirst into that New York strip steak. "Find out beforehand what the portion size is, then decide what you're going to eat," says Jody Mortenson, executive director of research and development for Friday's Hospitality Worldwide. "That steak could be 12 to 14 ounces. I know I only need 3 ounces of protein, so I'd ask for an extra plate and share."

Make your own fixings. Your fajita is still sizzling and now you, too, are starting to sweat, faced with enough guacamole, sour cream, and cheese to binge on for a week. Don't let the temptation even get to your table, says Mortenson. "I ask for mine without 'all the good stuff,' which happens to be the expensive stuff, so restaurants are happy to comply. A good substitution in my opinion is pico de gallo, which is tomatoes, onions, cilantro, and jalapeño peppers. Lettuce is also good for that extra crunch and flavor."

Know thy order. Everyone has ordered but you—and they're all staring. Flustered, you quickly point to the Vegetarian Bandito and turn in your menu. You feel great about your choice; that is, until it arrives, hidden under gobs of cheese.

That's not uncommon, warns Ziegler. "And many vegetarian entrées are made with cream cheese—not nonfat or low-fat cream cheese, but regular—to give them a little more zip." To keep it low-fat, hold the cheese or order a soy entrée, if they have one, like a soy-based meat alternative, she suggests.

Question all that glitters. A lot of chains brush butter on otherwise healthy, grilled items, says Mortenson. "It gives the perception to the guest that it's a juicy, moist, flavorful piece of meat," she adds. Just remind your waitress that you're ordering that low-fat entrée for a reason and have them hold the butter.

Take your time. Don't let the rest of the family rush you. "Eat slowly so your body and brain can connect and you know when you're full," says Ziegler.

Drop the fork. You don't have to clean your plate. Ask the waiter to take it away and put it in a doggie bag. "The sooner you do that, the less likely you are to pick at it when you're not really hungry," says Ziegler.

One note: "If you do choose to take it home, perishable food should not be kept at room temperature for longer than 3 hours," says Carolyn Raab, R.D., Ph.D., food and nutrition specialist for the Oregon State University Extension Service in Corvallis, who specializes in food safety.

Ending It Sweetly

Just when you thought the potential for damage was over, the grandkids start banging their fists on the table and chanting "dessert." Here are some tips for taming your sweet tooth.

Distract yourself. You're stuck at the table for another half-hour while the kids visit the sundae bar. Enjoy a cup of coffee or some hot spiced tea. "For me, it's a closure to the meal, and it gives me something to do with my hands while someone else is eating," says Dr. Raab. But be careful what you add. After-dinner drinks made with cream or liquor can have as many calories as a slice of cheesecake.

Go fruity. See if that hankering for something sweet can be satisfied by fruit. "Sometimes there's a fruit dessert like strawberries with cream—just have them hold the cream," suggests Ziegler. "Or get a fruit ice or sorbet, which are usually a small serving size."

Sherbet may be a better choice than the ice cream offered in most restaurants, which is usually top-of-the-line and has more calories and fat, says Dr. Raab. Low-fat frozen yogurt is also a good option.

Indulge a little. Truth be told, you won't balloon up if you have just a few bites. If some chocolate will send you out the door a happier person, treat yourself and split a dessert with the family. "That way, you get just enough to be satisfied," says Dr. Raab.

"There's room for all foods in your diet. Moderation is the key," adds Ziegler.

Party Time!

Your Guide to Eating for Entertainment

Call it the Golden Rule of Good Times: Where there's fun, there's food. After all, can you imagine a birthday without cake? The Fourth of July without burgers and hot dogs? The movies without popcorn?

Of course, the Golden Rule of Good Times has led to the Axiom for Amplified Appetites: When you're socializing and you're surrounded by food, you're more inclined to eat too much. So should you throw out your social calendar and turn down all invitations to special events for fear that you might overindulge?

No. Nothing's wrong with treating yourself once in a while. Let's face it: We like eating. We derive pleasure from it. And that's okay, as long as we indulge without *over*indulging.

It is possible to enjoy a holiday dinner, a tailgate party, or a night out on the town without guilt. Just remember the Law of Smart Partying: Eat, drink . . . and be wary.

Healthy Holidays

From Thanksgiving to New Year's, the 5-week winter holiday season can seem like one long, continuous feast. In fact, 69 percent of the people participating in a joint CNN/*Prevention* magazine survey revealed that they pretty much eat whatever they want during the holidays. And 40 percent said that they expect to gain weight as a result of their dietary lassitude.

For the average person, that means packing on 5 to 7 pounds, according to Jo Ann Carson, R.D., program director of clinical dietetics at the School of Allied Health Sciences at the University of Texas Southwestern Medical Center at Dallas. If that seems like a lot for such a short amount of time, think of it this way: To gain 5 pounds, you have to consume 17,500 extra calories over the 35 days between Thanksgiving and New Year's. That's 500 extra calories a day—a cinch for most of us.

It's not just that food is an ever-present temptation at this time of year. It's also that the holidays are emotionally charged times. "We're socializing with our relatives and friends and paying less attention to what we're eating," says Barbara Whedon, R.D., dietitian and nutrition counselor at Thomas Jefferson University Hospital in Philadelphia. "And there's constant pressure to eat—we don't want to offend the host by not trying her best recipe."

Considering the circumstances, you'd need all the willpower in the world to not give in to the urge to nosh. Relax—and cut yourself some slack. You can get through any holiday with your healthy eating habits intact if you keep these tips in mind, say experts.

Fill up beforehand. Your mom has her usual spread planned for Thanksgiving dinner. So you decide to make room for the impending feast by skipping breakfast—and maybe even lunch. Bad idea. All you're doing is making yourself ravenous. By the time you sit down, you could eat the entire turkey yourself—and maybe even the platter it's sitting on.

A much better option is to eat something before the big event, Whedon says. A carbohydrate-rich snack—a piece of fruit, a slice of bread, even a small plate of pasta—can quiet hunger pangs especially well. With your stomach no longer calling the shots, you can make healthier food choices.

Hit the (water) bottle. Another extremely effective appetite suppressant is good ol' H_2O. In fact, what you perceive as hunger may be thirst in disguise. Experts advise drinking at least eight 8-ounce glasses of water a day. But you may want to slurp down a few more when a big meal is in your future.

Gravitate toward veggies. Holiday meals usually feature a cornucopia of vegetable side dishes. Give these foods star billing on your plate. They'll fill you up, so you won't have a hankering for fattier fare. Just make sure that the ones you choose aren't swimming in butter or dripping with cheese sauce.

Occupy your plate. Leave something on your plate at all times. It serves as a signal to your host that you're so full you can't even finish what you have on your plate. That way, she won't try to foist more food on you—and you won't feel guilty for saying no. Just make sure that your decoy dish is something you don't particularly care for, so you don't keep nibbling away at it.

Excuse yourself. When you're finished eating, get up from the table. "Sitting in close proximity to food is much too tempting. It's your cue to eat," explains Susan Olson, Ph.D., clinical psychologist and weight-management consultant in Seattle and author of *Keeping It Off: Winning at Weight Loss*. Put some distance between yourself and all those goodies. And when you do, occupy yourself with something you enjoy, so you don't wander back to the table out of sheer boredom.

A Party Primer

Mention "party," and what comes to mind? Food and booze. Usually, there's an abundance of both. When everyone around you is mingling bites of cocktail wee-nies, chicken nuggets, and chips 'n' dip with sips of their favorite alcoholic beverages, it's mighty hard not to join in on the feeding frenzy.

Too often, eating and drinking become the focal point of a party. This is especially true when you don't know many people. You may hover around the buffet or the bar because you feel more comfortable there.

Remember, parties are for socializing and schmoozing. Try to eat less and talk more. And stick with these foolproof strategies suggested by experts to navigate those sumptuous spreads.

Practice preemptive nibbling. "Never go to a party on an empty stomach," says Agnes Kolor, R.D., a Pearl River, New York, nutritionist who consulted for *The Oprah Winfrey Show*. Snack on a banana or pret-zels beforehand. That way, you won't feel like making an immediate beeline for the buffet. Make sure the pretzels are salt-free, though. The salty kind just makes you thirsty.

Make a contribution. Give your host a hand by offering to bring a dish. Then choose something that supports your healthy eating habits—maybe salsa and nonfat tortilla chips or a vegetable plate with yogurt dip. That way, you know you have something healthful to nibble on.

Favor fiber. Choosing fiber-rich foods from the

Smart Strategies for Social Butterflies

For those whose job requirements include wining and dining, any given week can include several receptions, dinner parties, and other food-focused events. Here are several strategies for navigating the gustatory gauntlet and coming out with healthful eating habits intact.

■ Eat something small but filling about an hour beforehand.

■ Drink a large glass of water to curb hunger when you arrive.

■ Allow yourself two "bad" foods—maybe a brownie and a high-fat hors d'oeuvre—so you don't feel like they're off-limits.

■ Stick with veggies and avoid the fried hors d'oeuvres.

■ Finish your dinner salad, and ask for the dressing on the side.

■ Order healthier red wine or a wine spritzer, and avoid cocktails.

■ Mix your own drink when you can to control the amount of alcohol.

■ Drink at least two glasses of water for every alcoholic beverage.

■ Go ahead and order that rich dessert, then take just two bites and leave the rest.

■ If there's dancing or some other physical activity going on, participate with gusto.

buffet has a couple of advantages. For starters, these foods fill you up, so you won't feel like going back for fattier fare. Also, they take a long time to chew. You'll eat more slowly, which gives you better portion control. Besides, experts recommend that you consume 20 to 30 grams of fiber a day, and this is an ideal way to ensure that you meet your quota.

Fruits and veggies like apples, pears, oranges, and carrots have lots of fiber, as do air-popped popcorn and beans of any kind.

Feel the heat. Fiery spices act as appetite suppressants, so you won't eat as much. And as a bonus, they speed up your metabolism, allowing you to burn up the calories from your food a little faster. Look on the buffet for condiments such as hot mustard, cocktail sauce, salsa, and horseradish. Or top a burger with jalapeño peppers.

Seek out special dishes. Bypass those mixed nuts—you can eat those anytime. Instead, sample foods that you get only once in a blue moon. Maybe your host makes out-of-this-world chocolate chip cookies or a guacamole dip that's to die for. Go ahead and give it a try. Just keep a rein on your portion.

Keep your distance. Once you've made your food choices, do your socializing away from the buffet table, advises Edith Howard Hogan, R.D., a dietitian in Washington, D.C., and a spokesperson for the American Dietetic Association. "Fill your plate once, taking small portions. Then walk away. Otherwise, it's too easy to keep nibbling."

"I tell people to never stand right beside the buffet table," agrees Kolor. "When you do, you're constantly eating. Your hand automatically reaches down—it's an unconscious motion. You have more control if you put your food on your plate and then move on."

Stash your plate. Once you've cleaned off your plate, put it aside for the cleanup crew. (Or, if it's disposable, throw it in the trash.) If you stand around holding it, it just becomes a magnet for more food.

Keep your hands full. You may feel more comfortable having something in your hand when you mingle—kind of like a security blanket. If that's the case, make it a glass of mineral water, tomato juice, or diet soda. This strategy has an added advantage: If your host sees that you're holding a drink, she won't try to push liquor and other high-calorie beverages on you.

How to Navigate Bars

It's one of the three great ironies of the entertainment world: Only one of the Beach Boys surfed. The Monkees didn't play guitar on their records. And Sam Malone, bartender for *Cheers*, didn't drink.

In the real world, bellying up to the bar is tricky business, and not just because of the extra calories supplied by alcohol.

Suppose you decide to join your coworkers for happy hour at a nearby pub. You start out with a beer, which gives you the munchies. So you reach for those super-salty nuts or pretzels, which make you thirsty. So you order another beer. And around and around you go, filling up on calories that have nothing to offer you, nutrient-wise.

With a little preparation and a lot of common sense, you won't get caught up in this nutritional vortex. Here's what you need to know before you hoist that first glass.

Don't go empty. You've heard this before, but it bears repeating: If you go out on an empty stomach, you're bound to eat more. And what you're eating won't win any nutrition awards: Buffalo wings, potato skins, corn chips, cheese, and so on.

"If you're heading out right after work, plan to have a snack around 4:00 P.M.," says Liz Applegate, Ph.D., nutrition lecturer at the University of California, Davis, and author of *Power Foods*. "Stop by the cafeteria and pick up an apple, a carton of yogurt—something low-fat. Don't set foot in a bar when you're starving."

Skip salty snacks. Pretzels, corn chips, nachos, and other salty selections only make you drink more than you intended. "Bars kind of play you, you know?" Kolor says. "You eat all of their salty foods, so you end up buying more of their drinks."

If you do get hungry, order something that doesn't have a lot of salt, such as cut-up vegetables.

Food and Flicks

A movie just isn't a movie unless you have something to munch on while you're watching it. It's almost as though buying a ticket to the world of film fiction automatically suspends nutrition reality, too.

When you think about it, though, you're usually only in the theater for about two hours. "You can go that long without food," says Sachiko St. Jeor, R.D., Ph.D., professor of clinical nutrition and director of the nutrition education and research program at the University of Nevada School of Medicine in Reno. "Get into watching the movie as a pure experience, without shoveling down food you can't see—or really enjoy."

If you must have food at your fingertips, remember these guidelines for making smart choices for cinema snacking.

Pick the right popcorn. Popcorn is the classic treat to munch on during a movie. But theaters prepare it in a number of different ways, some of which can wallop you with artery-clogging saturated fat or trans-fatty acids.

When one group of researchers analyzed popcorn from six cinema chains across the country, they found that an average large order of unbuttered kernels had 2 days' worth of heart-damaging fat. Add the mysterious butterlike flavoring, and you may as well eat nine McDonald's Quarter Pounders. No kidding.

Your best bet is the air-popped variety. Order it plain, and you can eat as much as you want. After all, you're getting loads of fiber.

If the theater you frequent makes its popcorn in oil, ask whether it's nonhydrogenated. It still carries a load of fat, but not the nasty trans-fatty acids.

Cotton to candy. Some confections are kinder to your heart—and to your waistline—than others. Choose those that have no or low fat, such as licorice, mints, caramels, hard candy, and jelly beans. Keep in mind, though, that you're still consuming calories—empty calories. These foods have virtually no nutritional value.

Eating on the Run

Strategies for Shoppers and Travelers

Eating healthfully would be so much easier if temptation weren't lurking around every corner. From the candy bar in the vending machine to the fast-food court at the mall, food beckons you and teases your senses into submission.

There are ways to outwit these edible enticements without relying on willpower to do it. And if you're genuinely hungry, you can find healthful foods amidst the cookies and cappuccinos, the nachos and nuts. You just have to know what to look for.

Vending Machines: Hit the Jackpot

Buying food from a vending machine is kind of like playing a slot machine. Since you can't read the labels, you have no idea what you're getting, nutrition-wise. So you drop in your change, pull the lever, and hope for the best.

"Vending machines do offer better selections these days. But they tend to have their problems, too," says Edith Howard Hogan, R.D., a dietitian in Washington, D.C., and a spokesperson for the American Dietetic Association. If your choice is limited to candy bars and potato chips, for instance, it's not much of a choice at all. Either way, you're going to get between 10 and 25 grams of fat.

Your best bets: Look for fresh fruit, fruit juice, single-serving boxes of cereal, and pop-top single-serving cans of tuna, Hogan says. If none of these is available, then pretzels are a good low-fat, low-calorie option.

Convenience Stores: Good to Go

Once considered bastions of nutritionally vacant foods, 28 percent of all convenience stores now stock some sort of produce, according to the National Association of Convenience Stores.

Still, keep your guard up when browsing convenience-store aisles. You're going to encounter lots of high-fat, high-calorie grab-and-eat foods, says Liz Applegate, Ph.D., nutrition lecturer at the University of California, Davis, and author of *Power Foods*.

Your best bets: If you just want a snack, Dr. Applegate suggests pretzels or low-fat fig bars. For something more substantive, like a sandwich or burger, choose the least expensive one on the menu. It usually contains less meat—and less fat. Wash it down with orange or grape juice for an extra dose of vitamin C.

If you're buying something for the road, steer clear of the mega-bags of snack foods. They make it almost impossible to exercise any portion control.

Malls: Nutrition-Wise Selections

Perusing the food court at the local mall, you may think you've entered the land of giants. Who else could possibly eat those humongous soft pretzels, cookies, and hot dogs?

Truth be told, those tantalizing aromas are pretty darn hard to resist. And many of us do eat the whole thing—probably more often than we'd care to admit.

You may already suspect that these "monster foods" also pack monster doses of calories and fat. So here's the bad news: A giant-size order of nachos supplies 1,650 calories and 110 grams of fat. A giant-size muffin antes up 705 calories and almost 30 grams of fat. We could go on, but you get the idea.

To minimize mall munchies, eat *before* you shop. If you fill your stomach first, you're less likely to succumb to the sight and smell of foods, explains Michele Tuttle, R.D., former director of consumer affairs for the Food Marketing Institute in Washington, D.C.

Your best bets: Some mall café chains offer made-to-order sandwiches, which gives you control over what goes in them. At Au Bon Pain, for instance, you can choose from healthful fixin's such as smoked turkey, romaine lettuce, tomatoes, roasted red peppers, red onions, and whole-grain breads.

If you want something more "snackish," frozen yogurt is a refreshing treat. Both Friendly's and TCBY sell nonfat and low-fat varieties that range from 100 to 134 calories per serving.

Can't resist those cinnamon buns? You'll be happy to know that Cinnabon has introduced the "minibon delight," a reduced-fat cinnamon roll that contains about one-third of the calories (260) and one-quarter of the fat (6.5 grams) of the "classic" cinnamon roll.

Airlines: First-Class Fare

Airplane food has long been the butt of, pardon the pun, tasteless jokes. But consumer demand and competition among airlines is driving a shift toward better, more healthful in-flight meals.

Most airlines now offer their passengers a variety of special meals, including diabetic, kosher, vegetarian, low-sodium, low-fat, low-cholesterol, Hindu, and Muslim. Swissair, for instance, has 24 different variations to choose from, while Delta has 19.

Most airlines require that you request special meals ahead of time. If you can, do it when you book your flight. But even without advance reservations, certain carriers, like American Airlines, can serve Weight Watchers frozen meals on request on its transcontinental flights.

Your best bets: Ask ahead of time if your flight includes a meal. If it doesn't, pack healthy snacks such as bagels, a piece of fruit or dried fruit, single-serving boxes of cereal, and nonfat or low-fat sliced cheese. Or take along a packet of instant soup (bean, lentil, or pea) and request hot water when the beverage cart goes by.

In addition, many hotels will furnish a boxed lunch at a guest's request. Give room service a call to find out if you can get "one for the road."

Just remember to avoid cantaloupe, watermelon, carbonated drinks, and other gas-causing foods before or during a flight, says Maria Simonson, Sc.D., Ph.D., professor emeritus and director of the health, weight, and stress clinic at Johns Hopkins Medical Institutions in Baltimore. Otherwise, you can develop a painful gas bubble in your gastrointestinal tract from the change in altitude.

Remember, too, to drink lots of water—at least one glass for every hour that you're flying, Hogan advises. You can lose more than a pint of water through your skin and through breathing during a 3-hour flight.

Index

Underscored references indicate boxed text.

T